Surgery at a Glance

Surgery at a Glance

Vishal Jain MD
AIIMS, New Delhi
Ashish Jain MD
Medical College, Baroda

PEEPEE
PUBLISHERS and DISTRIBUTORS (P) LTD.

Surgery at a Glance

Published by
Pawaninder P. Vij
Peepee Publishers and Distributors (P) Ltd.
160, Shakti Vihar, Pitam Pura
Delhi - 110034 (India)
Ph: 27020004, 9811156083
e-mail: peepee160@yahoo.co.in

First Edition: **2004**

ISBN 81-88867-04-7

Printed at
Lordson, C-5/19, Rana Pratap Bagh, Delhi - 110 007

This Book is dedicated to
our
Parents
and
Best friends,
Arnab and Swarna

Preface

This handbook is an attempt to provide an answer to the vexed question "what should I read to get maximum output with optimum efforts"? This is one question, which confronts each and every medical student. This is my genuine effort to make learning and reading Surgery a simpleton task.

A well reasoned and relevant Anatomy and Pathophysiology has been included in each chapter to make the topic more comprehensive and memorizable. A list of differential diagnosis is included in each topic as an effort, towards broadening the horizon of knowledge. Diagnostic and Prognostic significances have been dealt elaborately.

Newer and emerging topics like Laparoscopic Techniques, Minimal Invasive Surgery; Pediatric Surgery and Cosmetic Surgery are written in a simpler and elusive way.

I think that this book will serve as the best companion for all the Final MBBS students, Interns and all those taking MD/MS entrance examinations.

Hope you will acknowledge my effort and encourage me to improve my writings in future.

Vishal Jain
Ashish Jain

Acknowledgement

We would like to express heartful regards to our parents for their constant support and encouragement whenever and wherever needed.

We deeply acknowledge help rendered by our friends like Biplab, Mohit, Lokesh, Navin, Rabha Balleb, Rohit, Randhir, and Mukesh. We would also like to thank Mr. Pawaninder P Vij of Pee Pee Publishers and Distributors (P) Ltd. for their expertise and help in bringing excellent book.

Vishal Jain
Ashish Jain

Contents

Chapter

1

General Surgery

BASIC KNOWLEDGE

Postoperative complications

Postoperative complications are clearly strongly dependent upon the type of surgery undertaken; no complication should be managed without the patient's history in mind. However, there are a number of common denominators, which are discussed here

Postoperative complications (general, early)

- **Pyrexia**
- Paralytic ileus
- Secondary haemorrhage often as a result of infection
- **Pneumonia**
- Wound or anastomosis dehiscence
- Deep venous thrombosis
- Urinary retention
- Urinary tract infection
- **Wound infection**
- Bowel obstruction due to fibrinous adhesions
- Confusion

PYREXIA

Fever in days 0-2

Causes include:

- Mild pyrexia
  - tissue damage and necrosis of the } at the site
  - haematoma } operation

- Higher persistent pyrexia
  - postoperative atelectasis (an Important cause)
  - specific infections related to the surgery
    - § biliary infection after biliary surgery
    - § urinary tract infection after urological surgery

Note that fever due to a blood transfusion may occur in this initial postoperative period.

Fever in days 3-5

Causes include:

- Bronchopneumonia
- Developing sepsis, which may be:
  - wound infection
  - drip site or drain infection
  - abscess formation, for example subphrenic o r pelvic, depending on the type of surgery performed.

Fever in days 5-7

Causes include:

- Venous thrombosis, in the limbs or pelvis
- Causes relating to specific operations, for example the failure of a bowel anastomosis, with fistula formation and leakage

Fever after the first week

Causes are less likely to be directly related to the specific operation undertaken.

Causes include:

- Wound sepsis
- Distant sites of sepsis eg cerebral or hepatic abscess
- Thrombotic disease

Preoperative Care

Preoperative care may be considered in terms of psychological and physical preparation of the patient for surgery.

Psychological preparation involves informing and obtaining written consent for the procedure and allaying any unneccessary fears that the patient may have.

Physical Preparation Involves

- Ensuring that the patient's diagnosis is correct and that symptoms have not changed.
- Assessment of the anaesthetic risks
- Making sure that the patient is as fit as possible

A thorough history and examination should be carried out, with an appropriate focus on operative and anaesthetic risk factors. Cardiovascular and respiratory fitness should be considered, as should any pre-existing medical condition, allergy or drug therapy including any oral contraceptive. Previous medical and anaesthetic history should be elicited and if surgery is to be postponed, it may be appropriate to give advice about losing weight, stopping smoking or reducing alcohol consumption.

Carry out the clinically indicated tests and then ensure that the patient is optimal for theatre i.e. he/she has been fasted, is well hydrated or has had necessary bowel or skin preparation etc.

Preoperative Tests

Preoperative tests should be performed where clinically indicated, and the results should be available before the patient goes to theatre.

- Urea, creatinine, electrolytes, full blood count and blood glucose BM testing shold be carried out in most patients
- Crossmatch or Group and Save blood as required by the operation.
- Specific blood tests:
  - liver function tests in Jaundice, alcohol abuse or malignancy
  - amylase in acute abdominal pain
  - blood Glucose in diabetic patients

  - clotting studies in liver disease or if on anticoagulants
  - thyroid function tests in thyroid disease
  - sickle cell tests in those from at-risk groups
- Chest X ray—if indicated
- ECG—if indicated

POSTOPERATIVE COMPLICATIONS (SPECIFIC)

Complications of Biliary Surgery

These complications of biliary surgery include:
- Retained stone in the bile duct
- Biliary peritonitis
- Bile duct damage
- Haemorrhage - the cystic and hepatic arteries and the liver bed are all vulnerable to operative trauma and may bleed heavily
- Complications of pre-existing jaundice
- Wound infection or abscess
- Ascending cholangitis
- Intraperitoneal abscess in the gallbladder bed and around the liver
- Chest infections

Complications of Subtotal Thyroidectomy

These are discussed in terms of:
- **Peroperative**
- **Immediate** postoperativehaemorrhage may present as rapid swelling of the neck, or as a large blood loss via the wound drain. A mediastinal haemorrhage may present as hypovolaemic shock.
- Laryngeal oedema—presents as acute airway obstruction
- Thyrotoxic crisis
- Hypocalcaemia—usually transient
- **Late postoperative**
- **Long term**

Complications of TURP

Immediate—within 48 hours:

- Primary haemorrhage
- Septicaemia
- Cardiovascular disturbance due to blood loss, transfusion
- Electrolyte imbalance, particularly hyponatraemia, from excessive absorption of irrigant-"TUR" syndrome

Intermediate - within 14 days:

- Secondary haemorrhage
- Urinary tract infection
- Chest infection
- Deep vein thrombosis and pulmonary embolism

Late:

- Urinary incontinence—from permanent damage to bladder sphincter
- Retrograde ejaculation—from disruption of the mechanism at the bladder neck that normally prevents entrance of semen into bladder during ejaculation; erection and orgasm are unaffected
- Bladder neck contracture
- Urethral stricture

Complications of Breast Surgery

- Psychological and social adjustment
- Arm oedema
- Skin necrosis
- Recurrence

Complications of Arterial Surgery

These include:

- Haemorrhage
- Thrombosis
- Embolism
- False aneurysm formation

Also complications of generalized arteriopathy e.g. stroke, myocardial ischaemia, intestinal ischaemia, renal failure.

Complications of Splenectomy

Early complications include:

- infection:
  - often subphrenic
- thrombosis:
  - a result of transiently raised platelet levels
  - patients are treated prophylactically with aspirin

Late complications are usually infective:

- Asplenic patients are susceptible to rapidly progressive pneumococcal and meningococcal infections
- The risk of infection is reduced by proper prophylaxis
- In children, elective splenectomy should be delayed until the immune system has matured; it is inadvisable to perform splenectomy before the age of five, and best to wait until age ten

Complications of Gastrectomy

It is important to elicit a history of gastrectomy since it may explain subsequent complications such as:

- Rapid feeling of fullness - very common but tends to improve over the first few months
- Bilious vomiting—varies in severity and persistence
- anaemia—iron deficiency or vitamin B12 deficiency
- Dumping
- Bolus obstruction of the gastric outlet stoma
- Diarrhoea or steatorrhoea
- 'blind loop syndrome' - a complication of a Polya gastrectomy due to bacterial overgrowth in the blind ended loop
- Weight loss—due to malabsorption and the above factors
- Osteomalacia—due to calcium and vitamin D malabsorption
- Ulceration—recurrent ulceration of the gastric remnant or stomal origin - in about 1% of cases
- Increased risk of subsequent gastric malignancy

Chapter 2

Head and Neck Diseases and Conditions

ACUTE EPIGLOTTITIS

Acute epiglottitis is the result of localized infection of the supraglottic larynx, usually by Haemophilus influenzae. This results in swelling of the epiglottis that obstructs the laryngeal inlet. Affects principally the pediatric age group(usually 1-5 years), but occasionally, if not rarely, seen in adults. Males seem to be more vulnerable than females in 4:1 ratio.If there is suspicion of acute epiglottitis the child should be admitted immediately because of the danger of airway obstruction.

The possible clinical features in paediatric age group includes :

- Croup occurs in a younger child - 2 or under
- Unwell; grey in colour - the child looks septic
- Voice is muffled, not hoarse
- If the child coughs it may sound like a "quack"
- Child is quiet and terrified
- Increasing dysphagia
- Drooling
- Stridor - of rapid onset and the child will prefer to sit upright and lean slightly forwards in an attempt to maintain the airway. The stridor may be fairly quiet.

In adults, possible clinical features may be severe pain that is worse on swallowing

Acute epiglotitis is a paediatric emergency. Management and treatment is as follows.

DO NOT

- Panic
- Alarm the parents or child
- Examine the child in any way - especially do not try to visualize the epiglottitis using a tongue depressor

DO

- Call a senior anaesthetist, paediatrician and ENT surgeon
- Alert theatres or ICU; the child needs to be admitted immediately

If respiratory arrest appears to be intervening before the senior help arrives, nebulised adrenaline can be used; this buys time but does not solve the underlying problem.

Immediate Management

- Admit immediately to hospital
- Don't give antibiotics
- Arrange a senior anaesthetist to intubate the patient and an ENT surgeon to perform a tracheostomy if needed
- Nebulised adrenaline can be used
- Be prepared to do an emergency laryngotomy in case of obstruction

Early Management

- The child is anaesthetised without using paralysing agent which may abolish the remaining airway. An inhalational anaesthetic is used
- The child is then examined by direct laryngoscopy and intubated if necessary
- If the airway cannot be secured then an ENT surgeon may have to perform an emergency tracheostomy

- blood samples and swabs are taken at this stage
- *Eradication of Bacteria*

  Broad-spectrum antibiotics – given IM initially while the IV set-up is being prepared, then IV for about a week, and shifted to oral route for the next 10 days.
  1. Ampicillin (200-400 mg/kg/day every 6 hours)
  2. Chloramphenicol (50-100 mg/kg/day every 6 hours)

ADENOID HYPERTROPHY

The adenoids are situated on the posterior wall of the nasopharynx in young children.

They begin to atrophy at about 6 years of age and have disappeared completely by the age of about 15.

However if a young child - between 1 and 4 years - suffers recurrent upper respiratory tract infection they may hypertrophy and become symptomatic because of consequent nasal and eustachian tube obstruction.

Treatment is adenoidectomy.

GLOBUS PHARYNGEUS

Globus pharyngis is the term applied to the sensation of a lump or discomfort in the throat. The condition is probably due to cricopharyngeal spasm occuring during moment of tension.

Discomfort may be relieved by eating and there is no interference with the swallowing of foods or liquids. Discomfort may be aggravated by the patient's constant action of swallowing. Also frequent introspection and anxiety seem to make the problem worse.

Note that some patients with globus pharyngis may be found to have reflux oesophagitis or a gastric ulcer and therefore a barium swallow may be performed to attempt to exclude organic pathology.

If discomfort persists then oesophagoscopy is essential.

RETROPHARYNGEAL ABSCESS

Retropharyngeal abscess is usually seen in infants or young children.

It may be caused by an upper respiratory tract infection that then causes an adenitis. The adenitis, which is in the retropharyngeal nodes, suppurates and forms an abscess.

The abscess is limited to one side of the midline. This is because of the intervening median raphe of the bucco-pharyngeal fascia which is firmly attached to the pre-vertebral fascia.

SALIVARY GLAND DISEASE

Salivary Gland Calculi

Sialolithiases are calcified stones which deposit in the salivary glands. They obstruct salivary outflow and predispose to infection. The submandibular gland is involved in 85% of cases, the parotid in about 10-15%, the sublingual gland in about 1%, and minor salivary glands in the remainder. They do not arise in the lingual or minor salivary glands.

They are composed of inorganic calcium and sodium phosphate salts mixed with mucous and cellular debris. They are radio-opaque and may be visualised on intraoral radiographs. Submandibular calculi tend to be large and single; those in the parotid, small and multiple.

The aetiology of salivary calculi is not known, but the submandibular gland is thought to be more vulnerable because of its more viscid secretion and elongated duct.

Submandibular calculi are common because stasis in the duct is encouraged both by the submandibular glands lying below the opening of the duct on the floor of the mouth, and the large mucous content of the secretions of the submandibular gland. They may be found anywhere along Warthin's duct, including its course within the gland.

Most occur in young to middle-aged adults, and they are rare in young children. Males and females are equally affected.

They should be differentiated from a stenosis of the duct orifice due to repeated trauma and fibrosis, e.g. following irritation from a sharp tooth, or a bite of the cheek.

Investigations

Physical exam including:
- Palpate the glands (diffusely swollen)
- Palpate the ducts (may palpate a stone)
  - Use bimanual palpation in the floor of the mouth
  - Milk saliva from duct-typically turbid and low volume

Imaging

- Plain films (occlusal for submandibular gland is best) may show calculi
  - 90% of submandibular calculi are radiopaque
  - 90% of parotid calculi are radiolucent
- Differentiate from phleboliths (round, laminated, multiple)
- Sialography
- Ultrasound
- CT scan (more sensitive)

Treatment Modalities

Stones in the anterior two-thirds of the submandibular duct in the floor of the mouth are removed by ductal dilation and massage. A suture is placed around the duct behind the stone so as to lift the duct upwards and prevent the stone from falling back out of reach. The stone is lifted out after making a longitudinal incision in the duct.

Stones in the hilum of the submandibular gland require excision of the gland because of their inaccessibility and the postoperative tendency for simple stone removal to result in stricture. Care must be taken to avoid damage to the mandibular branch of the facial nerve.

Chapter 3

Parathyroid Diseases

HYPOPARATHYROIDISM

Hypoparathyroidism may arise whenever there is inadequate secretion of PTH or the hormone is biologically ineffective. Under these circumstances the diminished physiologic action of PTH on the kidney leads to hypocalcaemia and hyperphosphataemia. Reduced end-organ sensitivity to PTH may also induce hypoparathyroidism. A constellation of clinical changes is associated with hypoparathyroidism.

Aetiology

Parathyroid gland deficiency:

- *Primary deficiency:*
  - idiopathic/congenital pseudohypoparathyroidism
  - DiGeorge syndrome
- *Secondary deficiency:*
  - destruction during thyroid, parathyroid or laryngeal surgery; by far the most common cause
  - infiltration by iron in haemochromatosis or by metastases

Reduced secretory activity:

- Hypomagnesaemia-Mg necessary for PTH secretion
- Vitamin D excess

End organ resistance:

- Pseudohypoparathyroidism
- Hypomagnesaemia

Clinical Features

With milder expressions of the syndrome, the clinical manifestations are subtle. At the other extreme more overt expressions of acute hypocalcaemia may be present:

- Increased neuromuscular excitability:
  - may cause Chvostek's sign, tetany, carpopedal spasms, laryngeal stridor and convulsions
- Mental changes—ranging from irritability to depression and frank psychosis
- Neurological signs suggesting an intracranial tumour with elevated CSF pressure e.g. papillo-edema
- Intracranial calcification visualised by skull radiology—particularly, in the basal ganglia
- Calcification of lens, leading to formation of cataracts
- Abnormalities of cardiac conduction—mainly prolonged Q-T intervals and T-wave changes
- Abnormalities of dentition with defective enamel, dental hypoplasia, and delayed eruption of teeth
- Alopecia with premature greying
- Chronic mucocutaneous candidiasis is common in autoimmune

Investigations

Diagnosis is based on:

- Low serum calcium
- Increased plasma phosphate—low in hypocalcaemia due to intestinal malabsorption or vitamin D deficiency
- Normal alkaline phosphatase—raised in hypocalcaemia due to chronic renal failure
- Skull radiology may reveal basal ganglia calcification
- PTH: low plasma levels
- Urinary cAMP excretion rises following administration of PTH

Treatment

Acute symptomatic hypocalcaemia requires urgent correction with intravenous calcium; oral calcium is rarely adequate to sustain normocalcaemia.

Permanent hypoparathyroidism and pseudohypoparathyroidism are treated with supraphysiological doses of vitamin D or one of its active metabolites; the metabolites are preferred since they have a relatively short half life and permit easier modification of the treatment regime.

Doses of 1.25-2.5 mg per day of vitamin D are required.

Maintenance doses of the metabolites are:

- 0.5 to 1.0 mcg per day 1,25 (OH)2 D
- 1.0 to 2.0 mcg per day 1 OH D

Supplementary calcium is only required if the diet provides less than 600 mg per day

HYPERPARATHYROIDISM

Hyperparathyroidism is a condition in which there is excessive secretion of parathyroid hormone. The principal target organs are the kidney and bone, with a secondary effect on the gut through 1,25 dihydroxy vitamin D.

Hyperparathyroidism can be primary, secondary or tertiary according to the extent of excessive parathyroid hormone produced, and the degree of autonomy of the parathyroid glands.

Clinically, there may be effects of both hypercalcaemia and of hypocalcaemia.

Investigations should include serum calcium and phosphate, and parathyroid hormone.

PRIMARY HYPERPARATHYROIDISM

This may be defined as a circulating level of PTH which is inappropriately high for the prevailing level of calcium. Most patients are hypercalcaemic but the condition may equally occur in normocalcaemic patients with co-existent vitamin D deficiency. It implies hyperfunction of one or more parathyroid glands with a change in the set point for the control of calcium.

It has an incidence of 0.5 per 1000 and is most common between 40 and 60 years of age when it is twice as common in women than men. In other age groups, the sex incidence is roughly equal. In young people of either sex, it is important to investigate possible multiple endocrine neoplasia.

Aetiology

Over 80% of primary hyperparathyroidism cases are caused by a single parathyroid adenoma of the chief or clear cells of the parathyroid gland.

Other causes include:

- Multiple adenomas—5%
- Diffuse hyperplasia:
  - of chief cells—8%
  - of clear cells—4%
- Carcinoma—2%
- Ectopic PTH-secreting tumour

Co-existence of hypercalcaemia with hypertension and neurofibroma is suggestive of multiple endocrine neoplasia—MEN I or MEN IIa. Primary hyper-thyroidism is rarely familial.

Pathology

In hyperparathyroidism, the principally affected sites are where the bone turnover is most active, for example the trabecular bone of the vertebrae, the phalanges, the ends of long bones and parts of the skull.

Macroscopically there is demineralisation of bone. Increased bone reabsorption leads to subperiosteal resorption of the phalanges, thinning of the cortex, and the formation of bone cysts or brown tumours. Deformities can lead to fracture or bending.

Microscopically there is an increased number of osteoclasts which increase the amount of bone resorption. The marrow spaces are filled with fibrous tissue producing osteitis fibrosa.

The increased osteoblast activity causes an increased woven-non-lamellar–bone trabeculae.

Clinical Features

"Bones, moans and stones" is the classical description of hyperparathyroidism but such clear cases are uncommon.

Clinical features due to excess PTH may include:

- Bone resorption leading to bone pain, pathological fracture, and rarely, osteitis fibrosa cystica; characteristic changes visible on radiography
- Renal calculi occur in 10-15% of patients with primary hyperparathyroidism
- Other features of metastatic calcification may be present such as nephrocalcinosis, and corneal calcification; occasionally, chondrocalcinosis may be evident on radiology
- Rarely, primary hyperparathyroidism may present as acute pancreatitis
- Polyuria, thirst, weakness, vomiting

Features attributable to hypercalcaemia may be evident in primary and tertiary hyperparathyroidism.

- In secondary hyperparathyroidism, the clinical picture may be complicated by hypocalcaemia. In chronic renal failure, co-existent osteomalacia results in renal osteodystrophy.

Investigations

The investigations in primary hyperparathyroidism include:

- Raised serum Ca with high or normal—but inappropriately high for the level of Ca—serum PTH
- Serum alkaline phosphatase—often normal but may be markedly increased in bone disease
- Serum phosphate:

  - decreased in about half of cases
  - a raised serum phosphate suggests nonpara-thyroid hypercalcaemia
  - a normal serum phosphate is not diagnostically useful
- urine Ca—increased in most patients
- metabolic acidosis is reflected by reduced plasma bicarbonate and high plasma chloride
- bone radiographs abnormal—pathognomonic subperiosteal bone resorption of the phalanges; there may be loss of the lamina dura of the teeth; in severe cases osteitis fibrosa cystica is present
- ultrasound of the neck may reveal a thyroid parathyroid adenoma; also may be shown by a radioactive thallium technetium scan
- two-site radioimmunoassays for PTH can differentiate primary hyperparathyroidism—high PTH—from malignancy related hypercalcaemia (low PTH)
- venous PTH sampling—may be employed to localise the the source of the PTH on occasions where it has not been identified during initial surgery

Radiology

The radiological changes in hyperparathyroidism are:
- Classically, subperiosteal bone resorption—most often on the radial aspect of the middle phalanges of the fingers; the extent correlates well with the increased serum alkaline phosphatase
- Loss of lamina dura—the thin layer of compact bone forming the sheath for the tooth socket—a late sign
- Extensive bone resorption in the skull gives a stippled 'pepper pot' appearance
- Cystic lesions—brown tumours—may occur elsewhere in the skeleton—appear as rounded radiolucent lesions which are trabeculated—but are less common and a late sign

- Resorption of metaphyseal bone in children gives rise to crippling skeletal deformities
- There may be diffuse osteopenia

Treatment

For primary hyperparathyroidism, surgery is indicated in all patients under the age of 60 years and in other patients with a serum calcium concentration above 3.00 mmol per litre.

Treated patients may show a mild transient state of hypoparathyroidism for several days or weeks afterwards until the remaining previously suppressed glands recover. Mild circumoral and digital paraesthesiae may occur and are easily controlled using iv or oral calcium.

Severe and prolonged low serum levels of calcium, magnesium, and phosphate may occur postoperatively and require an active vitamin D metabolite such as 1 HCC.

SECONDARY HYPERPARATHYROIDISM

Secondary hyperparathyroidism refers to hyperplasia of all four parathyroid glands secondary to prolonged hypocalcaemia or hyperphosphataemia. It is a normal homeostatic response and is the most common form of hyperparathyroidism. Serum calcium levels are replenished from skeletal stores, and by increasing both renal tubular reabsorption and gut absorption of calcium

Aetiology

Secondary hyperparathyroidism is due to chronic hypocalcaemia associated with:

- Chronic renal failure—defective absorption of calcium in the gut due to reduced levels of 1, 25 dihydroxy cholcalciferol
- Malabsorption and vitamin D deficiency

Clinical Features

SAME AS THOSE IN PRIMARY HYPER-PARATHYROIDISM

Investigations

Investigations in secondary hyperparathyroidism show:

- Low or normal serum calcium
- PO4 is raised or normal in chronic renal failure; and lowered in malabsorption
- Serum alkaline phosphatase is elevated

Treatment

The aim in secondary hyperparathyroidism is to treat the underlying cause.

Skeletal calcium may be conserved by administering active metabolites of vitamin D such as:

- 1 hydroxy cholecalciferol—1 HCC—0.5-2.0 mcg per day
- 1,25 dihydroxy cholecalciferol—1,25 HCC—0.25-1.0 mcg per day

Both agents increase the intestinal absorption of calcium and directly inhibit the activity of parathyroid cells. Care is necessary to avoid precipitating hypercalcaemia.

TERTIARY HYPERPARATHYROIDISM

Tertiary hyperparathyroidism describes a condition in which autonomous parathyroid activity and hypercalcaemia occur following prolonged secondary hyperparathyroidism.

The set point at which serum calcium shuts off PTH production is raised. It is most commonly seen in patients undergoing maintenance renal dialysis. Tertiary hyperparathyroidism may also occur in patients with long standing malabsorption or chronic renal failure.

Associated Conditions

Tertiary hyperparathyroidism is associated with the following conditions:
- Renal dialysis
- Chronic renal failure
- Chronic malabsorption

Investigations

Investigations in tertiary hyperparathyroidism show:
- Raised Ca in the serum
- Albumin is normal or low
- PO4:
  - Decreased or normal in chronic renal failure
  - Decreased in malabsorption
- serum alkaline phosphatase is raised
- plasma PTH raised

Treatment

The intermittent administration of i.v. 1,25 (OH)2 D may postpone the evolution of secondary hyperparathyroidism to tertiary hyperparathyroidism.

The treatment of choice is subtotal parathyroidectomy leaving about 100 mg of parathyroid tissue. The tissue may be implanted into the arm or another accessible site to facilitate future surgery if required. Invasive tumour like overgrowth of the implants may occu

PSEUDOHYPOPARATHYROIDISM

Pseudohypoparathyroidism is a rare disorder characterised by failure of target cells to respond to parathyroid hormone. It is inherited in an autosomal dominant fashion.

Features are similar to hypoparathyroidism.

There is peripheral resistance to the action of PTH.

Classification

There are two main types of pseudohypoparathyroidism:

- *Type I:*
  - adenylate cyclase is not activated by PTH
  - urinary cAMP levels do not rise when PTH is administered
- *Type II:*
  - cells fail to respond to the intracellular cAMP signal
  - urinary cAMP levels rise when PTH is administered

Clinical Features

There are the usual clinical features of hypocalcaemia:

- Carpopedal spasm
- Paraesthesiae
- Abdominal cramps
- Papilloedema
- Epilepsy

Associated endocrine disorders include:

- Hypothyroidism
- Diabetes mellitus

Phenotypically pseudohypoparathyroidism is associated with:

- Short stature
- Mental retardation
- Obesity
- Strabismus
- Subcutaneous calcification—rare in acquired hypoparathyroidism
- Shortened metacarpals and metatarsals:
  - o Brachydactyly
  - o Especially 3rd, 4th and 5th rays
- Bowing of the legs
- Rounded moon face
- Cerebral calcification

Metacarpal shortening may easily be demonstrated by asking the patient to make a fist and observing that the relevant knuckles are absent.

Investigations

The laboratory results show:

- Low serum calcium
- increased plasma phosphate—low in Hypocalcaemia due to intestinal malabsorption or vitamin D deficiency
- Normal alkaline phosphatase—raised in hypocalcaemia due to chronic renal failure
- skull radiology may reveal basal ganglia calcification
- high PTH concentrations
- In type I pseudohypoparathyroidism, urinary cAMP fails to rise following administration of PTH
- In type II pseudohypoparathyroidism, urinary cAMP rises normally following PTH administration

PSEUDOPSEUDOHYPOPARATHYROIDISM

This is used to describe patients whom present with the somatic abnormalities of pseudohypothyroidism but lack the biochemical ones.

The occurrence of pseudopseudohypoparathyroidism in the same families as pseudohypoparathyroidism has been reported. This may represent incomplete genetic expression of the same genetic abnormality.

Chapter 4

Thyroid Diseases and Conditions

HYPERTHYROIDISM

Thyrotoxicosis is a disease caused by excessive concentrations of free thyroid hormones (most often T4).

Many of the clinical features of thyrotoxicosis are characterised by signs of sympathetic overactivity such as tremor, tachycardia, and sweating producing weight loss, fatigue and heat intolerance.

The level of catecholamines is normal but the excess thyroid hormones seem to potentiate the action of the catecholamines.

Hyperthyroidism is extremely common, affecting perhaps 2 to 5% of all females at some time in their lives. The vast majority of cases are caused by intrinsic thyroid disease; a pituitary cause is extremely rare.

Aetiology

- Primary:
  - due to pathology within the thyroid gland
  - most common.
- Pecondary:
  - a pathological process causes excessive stimulation of a normal thyroid gland.

Hyperthyroidism (Primary)

This is hyperthyroidism secondary to pathology within the thyroid gland. Ninety perent of cases are due to:

- Grave's disease

- Toxic nodular goitre:
  - multinodular
  - single toxic nodule—usually an adenoma.

Other common causes:

- Thyroiditis
  - de Quervain's
  - silent/post-partum
  - Hashimoto's—hashitoxicosis may develop mid-course.

Uncommon:

- Intentional/factitious
- Overenthusiastic therapy
- Drug-induced
- Jod—Basedow.

Hyperthyroidism (Secondary)

Hyperthyroidism as a result of pathology in another organ which causes excess stimulation of the thyroid gland.

Excess TSH:

- Uncommon:
  - TSH secreting pituitary adenoma
  - pituitary stimulation due to excessive hypothalamic release of TRH.
- Rare:
  - hydatidiform moles
  - choriocarcinoma
  - embryonal testicular carcinoma.

Extraneous thyroid hormone—all rare:

- Struma ovarii—ovarian teratoma with thyroid tissue.
- Metastatic, well differentiated thyroid carcinoma.

Clinical Features of Hyperthyroidism

Typical presentations of thyrotoxicosis

- Increased heat production—warm, moist skin, heat intolerance.

- Telangiectasia, palmar erythema, pretibial myxo-edema, onycholysis.
- Weight loss, increased appetite, increased frequency of bowel movement but frank diarrhoea is uncommon; steatorrhoea may occur; dyspepsia; like juvenile-onset diabetes mellitus, may cause a decrease in weight despite an increased appetite.
- Oligomenorrhoea.
- Tachycardia, exertional dyspnoea, hyperdynamic circulation; systolic hypertension is common and diastolic hypertension can occur in up to 30% of patients.
- Tiredness, irritability, nervousness.
- Fine tremor, hyperkinesia.
- There are eye signs in Graves' disease.

Others:

- Occasionally, bone pain due to osteoporosis.
- In elderly patients, there may be atrial fibrillation or cardiac failure.
- Alopecia, pruritus, pretibial myxoedema, acro-pachy.

Atypical Presentations of Thyrotoxicosis

These may include:
- Atrial arrhythmias in middle aged patients.
- Severe proximal myopathy with normal CK values
- Deterioration or unmasking of myasthenia gravis
- Hypokalaemic periodic paralysis—especially in orientals.
- Chronic diarrhoea.
- Hypercalcaemia.
- Osteoporosis.
- gynaecomastia (Fig. 4.1).

Differential Diagnosis

The differential diagnosis of hyperthyroidism includes:
- Anxiety states:
  - differentiation may be difficult clinically

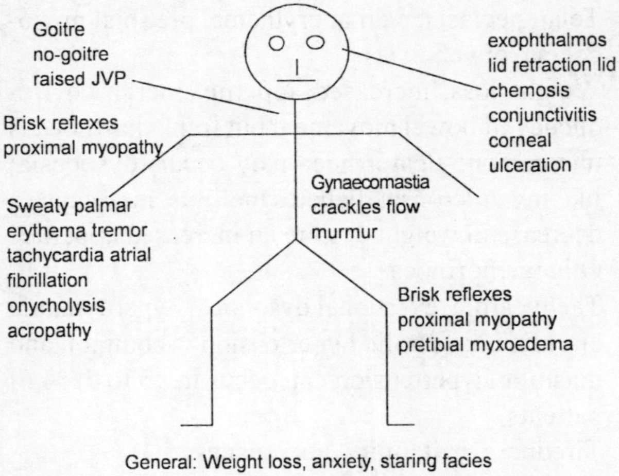

Fig. 4.1: Diagram of the clinical features of hyperthyroidism

- positive findings for thyrotoxicosis are eye signs, proximal myopathy, wasting, hyperdynamic circulation with warm peripheries
- anxiety tends to cause clammy hands.

• Phaeochromocytoma:
  - especially if the patient is hypertensive.

Investigations in Hyperthyroidism

Thyroid function tests consists of:
- T3 and T4 determination.
- TSH determination—normal serum TSH concentration nearly always excludes the diagnosis of thyrotoxicosis; the rare exceptions to this are a TSH-producing pituitary tumour or thyroid hormone resistance syndrome.
- TRH stimulation test (rarely performed)
- Radioisotope iodine scanning
- Serology.

Other investigations:
- FBC:
  - normochromic normocytic anaemia may be seen in Grave's disease.

- ESR:
  - raised in Grave's disease
  - high in subacute thyroiditis.
- calcium—often raised
- LFTs—may be abnormal in Grave's disease.

Treatment Modalities

There are three treatment options available:

- Drug treatment
- Surgery
- Radioiodine.

1. Drug treatment

- Beta blockers for acute symptomatic treatment.
- Antithyroid drugs for long term treatment
  - antithyroid drugs are prescribed either for the short-term control of thyrotoxicosis prior to definitive treatment, or in the hope of achieving remission in patients with Graves' disease, especially in those presenting under the age of 40. Generally a course of 18 months is recommended but the probability of achieving long-term remission is less than 50%.
  - rates of remission are lower in males, in older patients, and in those patients with severe hyperthyroidism.
  - antithyroid drugs are ineffective in thyroiditis (viral, postpartum or amiodarone induced)—this is because the action of the antithyroid drugs is to block production of thyroid hormones whereas the hyperthyroidism associated with thyroiditis is caused by release of stored thyroid hormone from damaged thyroid cells.

2. Surgical or radio-iodine treatment in thyrotoxicosis

Indications for radioiodine treatment include:

- Radio-iodine treatment.

- increasingly becoming the first-line treatment for adults with Graves' thyrotoxicosis.
- treatment of choice for most patients with relapsed Graves' disease.
- treatment of choice in patients with toxic nodular hyperthyroidism.
- women of child-bearing age are advised to avoid pregnancy for four months after receiving radio-iodine treatment.
- the presence of Graves' ophthalmopathy is a relative contra-indication to radio-iodine therapy because it may deteriorate after radio-iodine treatment.

Specific indications for surgical intervention include:

- Patient choice
- Large goitre that is unlikely to resolve with antithyroid drugs.

Pregnancy and Thyrotoxicosis

Pregnant women with hyperthyroidism require management by a hospital specialist.

Antithyroid drugs are the treatment of choice in pregnancy but the "block and replace" regime is contraindicated.

In North America propylthiouracil is preferred as it is excreted less in breast milk and carbimazole may be associated with aplasia cutis. 'The suggested association of carbimazole with neonatal aplasia cutis has led some clinicians to prefer propylthiouracil for use during pregnancy (2).'

The smallest dose of antithyroid medication possible should be used because of the risk of fetal hypothyroidism—carbimazole 5-10 mg/day; propylthiouracil 50-100 mg/day. Generally treatment is withdrawn 4 weeks prior to delivery after which normal doses may be resumed.

Often hyperthyroidism due to Graves' disease improves spontaneously across pregnancy, so a smaller dose of antithyroid drug may be required.

Radio-iodine is contraindicated and pregnancy should be avoided for at least 4 months following receipt of I-131.

THYROID EYE DISEASE

Ophthalmologic involvement is common in Graves' disease, and it accounts for the majority of dysthyroid eye disease. Typically, it develops within 12 months of the onset of hyperthyroidism but may precede it or develop concurrently with it.

Very rarely, dysthyroid eye disease may occur in the presence of autoimmune primary hypothyroidism.

Stimulating TSH receptor antibodies are inevitably found.

Fibroblastic deposition of glycosaminoglycans and lymphocytic infiltration into the extraocular muscles and retrobulbar connective tissue produces retrobulbar oedema. This is followed by fibrosis with restricted movement as the muscles become tethered to the surrounding structures.

Consequently:

- The eye is pushed forwards and there is axial proptosis The cornea may become exposed with drying, irritation and later ulceration.
- Extraocular muscle movement is impaired.
- Increasing pressure is exerted on the optic nerve with loss of acuity and eventually, atrophy.
- Venous drainage from the orbit is impaired resulting in conjunctival and periorbital oedema, and conjunctival injection.

Clinical Features

- 5-10% cases are unilateral.

Presentation may include:

- Orbital pain

- Lacrimation
- Photophobia
- Blurred or double vision.

Features found on examination may include:

- Proptosis—usually bilateral, often asymmetric; less commonly, symmetrical.
- Lid retraction and lid lag.
- Periorbital puffiness.
- Impaired extraocular muscle function.
- Chemosis—conjunctival oedema—and injection
- Exposure keratitis; possibly, corneal ulceration.
- Ophthalmoplegia—generally superior rectus producing diplopia maximal on upward and outward gaze.
- Reduced visual acuity.
- Papilloedema; optic atrophy.
- Pretibial dermopathy (the least common manifestation of Grave's disease) occurs in patients with severe ophthalmology—generally occurs as a nodular or diffuse thickening of the skin of the anterior lower leg, but it can occur elsewhere.

The management of dysthyroid eye disease can be divided into immediate and longterm management. The *immediate priorities* are to treat the endocrine disorder and render the patient euthyroid, prevent any visual loss and protect the cornea:

- Treatment of thyroid disease (although thyroid eye disease may occur before other signs of Graves' disease and does not always respond to treatment of thyroid disease); also thyroid eye disease may occur for the first time after hyperthyroidism treatment.
- Artificial tears are often required for lubrication
- eyelids can be taped closed or a lateral tarsorraphy can be undertaken (stitching the eyelids together at their outer corner).
- High dose steroids may facilitate medical decompression of the optic nerve (visual loss may occur

due to compression of the optic nerve, particularly when there is minimal exopthalmos. Optic nerve function should be assessed in terms of colour vision and the presence of any central scotomas).

- Guanethidine eye-drops may reduce lid retraction (often patient does not tolerate longterm treatment)
- Surgical decompression may be employed—this surgery utilises space in ethmoidal, sphenoidal and maxillary sinuses.
- Orbital radiotherapy—this treatment modality is increasingly utilised at an early stage in management of thyroid eye disease.
- A Fresnel prism stuck to one lens of a spectable may be used in the management of diplopia—this lens is changed with respect to changes in exophthalmus.

Longterm management aims to restore external ocular muscle function and restore appearance.

There is evidence that thyroid eye disease may occasionally be made worse by treatment with radioiodine (1).

Treatment with bromocriptine, somatostatin analogues, plasmapharesis and acupuncture have been suggested for the management of this condition but a role for these agents requires confirmation (1).

Note that thyroid-eye disease generally goes into spontaneous remission with time (1).

Neonatal Hyperthyroidism

This uncommon condition results from transplacental passage of stimulating IgG TSH-receptor antibodies to the infant from a mother with a past or current history of Graves' disease.

The maternal concentration of stimulating TSH-receptor antibodies must be high for the neonate to be affected and maternal pre-tibial myxoedema serves a useful marker of the maternal state.

Clinical Features

Presentation is with:

- Goitre
- Exophthalmus
- Failure to thrive
- Fever
- Often marked tachycardia and cardiac failure if treatment is delayed.

Treatment

The condition is often self-limiting since the maternal immunoglobulins have a half-life of about three weeks in the infant.

Short term treatment with carbimazole and propranolol may be life saving.

Thyroid function tests should be regularly monitored in affected babies.

THYROID CANCER

Thyroid carcinoma is rare, having an annual incidence of about 3-5 per 100,000.

Thyroid cancer accounts for about 0.4% of all cancer deaths. Women are affected more commonly than men in a ratio of 2-3:1.

Types

- Papillary adenocarcinoma : 60—80%
- Follicular adenocarcinoma : 20—25%
- Medullary adenocarcinoma : 5%
- Anaplastic carcinoma : 5%
- Thyroid lymphoma : <1%.

Aetiology

Little is known about the aetiology of thyroid cancer. Low dose radiation may be an important factor as many cases have been reported 10-30 years after X-ray exposure.

There is evidence that individuals treated with radioiodine have a small but significant increase in the incidence of thyroid cancer (1).

Clinical Features

A rapidly growing hard thyroid mass with lymphadenopathy and indicators of extrathyroidal invasion e.g. hoarseness, dysphagia is suggestive of maligancy. Other important factors to elicit are a history of exposure to ionizing radiation and a family history of thyroid cancer.

The exact presentation varies with the type of tumour for example:

- Papillary—very slow growth; often spreads to lymph nodes in the neck. The most common thyroid cancer.
- follicular—usually middle aged women. Often spread to bones and lungs.
- medullary—20% of cases associated with MEN-II; raised calcitonin, cervical nodes often affected; may present with intractable diarrhoea and flushing anaplastic—usually in older patient; may present with a firm rapidly growing.

Investigations

- Fine needle biopsy—the most effective method of distinguishing benign from malignant nodules. Results usually expressed as positive, suspicious, non-diagnostic or negative.
- Tumour products—basal and pentagastrin-stimulated serum calcitonin distinguishes medullary carcinoma. Serum thyroglobulin is non-diagnostic and may be found in benign and malignant lesions
- Ultrasound—not useful as a primary test but may help to distinguish cystic lesions—nearly always benign—from solid lesions.
- Thyroid scanning with radioiodine—thyroid cancer is characteristically a 'cold nodule' on radioisotope scanning of the thyroid; hot nodules rarely malignant. Not a primary test (Fig. 4.2).

Scintiscans of thyroid. The scan on the left is normal. A typical scan of a "cold" thyroid nodule failing to accumulate iodide isotope is shown on the right.

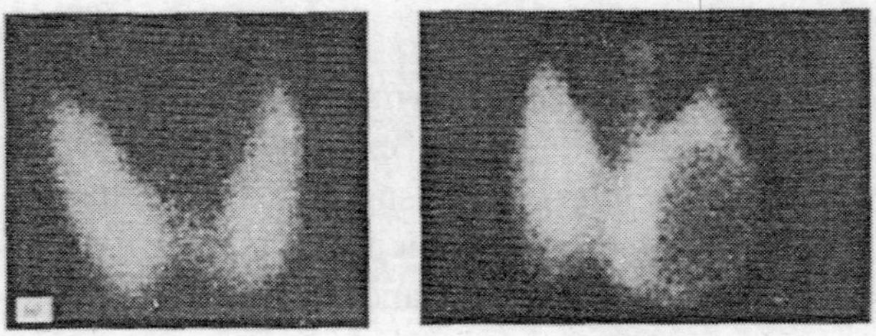

Fig. 4.2

- Chest X-ray—lung secondaries
- Thyroid mass, stridor, vocal

Management

Most thyroid tumours are treated surgically with follow up radioiodine ablation if the tumour will concentrate I^{131}.

Papillary and follicular tumours are usually treated by near total or total thyroidectomy. An ipsilateral total lobectomy and isthmusectomy is indicated if only one lobe is affected. Following surgery, most centres will then ablate all residual functioning thyroid tissue with radioactive iodine over a period of 6-12 months. Others would propose administering suppressive doses of thyroxine and monitoring the patient for possible recurrence but this has become less fashionable recently.

Medullary and anaplastic tumours do not generally take up I^{131} and are both treated by total thyroidectomy. Cervical lymph node dissection and external irradiation may also be performed.

Prognosis

Better differentiated tumours carry a better prognosis:

- Papillary—20 year survival is greater than 90% if the carcinoma is small and intrathyroidal. The prognosis is is slightly worse in the elderly where there is a greater tendency to more aggressive disease and lung metastasis in the form of lymphangitis carcinomatosa.

- Follicular—20 year survival is 60-70%. Angio-invasion is associated with greater mortality
- Medullary—20 year survival is 70-80%. Less differentiated variants have a poorer survival.
- Anaplastic—20 year survival is less than 5%. Most die within 1 year.

Urgent Referral for Suspected Thyroid Cancer

Urgent referral:

- Hoarseness that persists for more than 6 weeks
- Ulceration of oral mucosa that persists for more than 3 weeks.
- Oral swellings that persist for more than 3 weeks
- If there are red or red and white patches seen on examination of the oral mucosa.
- Dysphagia that persists for 3 weeks.
- Unilateral nasal obstruction especially when associated with purulent discharge.
- If there is unexplained tooth mobility that is not associated with periodontal disease.
- Unresolving neck masses for more than 3 weeks
- The presence of cranial neuropathies.
- An orbital mass or orbital masses.

The level of suspicion is further increased if the patient is a heavy alcohol drinker or heavy smoker and is aged over 45 years and male. The chewing of tobacco (called Gutkha in India) or the chewing of Paan Masala or Betel should also increase the level of suspicion.

1. Papillary Adenocarcinoma of the Thyroid

This is the most commonly recognised thyroid cancer and the most easily diagnosed by fine needle biopsy. It accounts for over 60% of thyroid carcinoma. Women are affected more often than men. Papillary carcinomas occur rather evenly from the third to seventh decade and account for 80% of all thyroid cancer in individuals under 40 years of age.

Histologically, it shows papillae around a fibro-vascular stalk and usually contains elements of follicular differentiation. It is slow growing and may be asymptomatic for many years. It is often multifocal. Local spread to regional nodes in the neck and mediastinum is common and 50% of patients show nodal metastases at the time of death.

It is not uncommon for a local lymph node metastasis to be detected before the primary tumour. Early metastases of this type have been termed "lateral aberrant thyroid".

Distant metastasis to the lungs or bone is rare.

2. Follicular Adenocarcinoma of the Thyroid

This accounts for 20-25% of thyroid cancer with females affected three times as frequently as males and with a peak incidence at 55 years of age. It is usually unifocal and rarely spreads to lymph nodes. It is angioinvasive to lungs and bone in over 50% of cases and this may be the first sign of malignancy.

It is a well differentiated tumour and shows reasonable response to TSH. It may take up iodine and may form thyroid hormones. Very rarely, it produces hyperthyroidism.

3. Medullary Adenocarcinoma of the Thyroid

This is a malignancy of the parafollicular cells of the thyroid.

This is a relatively uncommon thyroid carcinoma accounting for about 5% of thyroid malignancy. Both sexes are equally affected and the age of onset is variable. Aggressiveness is intermediate between that of well-differentiated and anaplastic lesions. About 80-90% of cases are sporadic; these usually affect adults and are unilateral. The other cases are familial, with an autosomal dominant inheritance; these tumours are typically bilateral and multifocal.

The medullary carcinoma arises from the para-follicular or C-cells of the thyroid which are of neural crest origin and form part of the APUD system. Calcitonin levels tend to be elevated and diagnostic. Levels of serum serotonin, ACTH and other peptides may also be raised. Spread to both regional lymph nodes and distant metastases to bone, liver and lung are common.

Diarrhoea and facial flushing are associated with medullary carcinomas of the thyroid.

Twenty percent of cases occur as part of the MEN-II syndrome.

4. Anaplastic Carcinoma of the Thyroid

This is seen most frequently in individuals over 60 years of age with an equal incidence in both sexes. It is an aggressive tumour which may arise from dedifferentiation of a papillary or follicular thyroid cancer. It accounts for about 5% of thyroid carcinomas.

Local invasion occurs to the trachea and to the oesophagous and the patient may present with dyspnoea or dysphagia respectively. Almost 80% of patients have a history of long-standing goitre.

Thyroid require total thyroidectomy and aggressive lymph node dissection.

Surgical Options

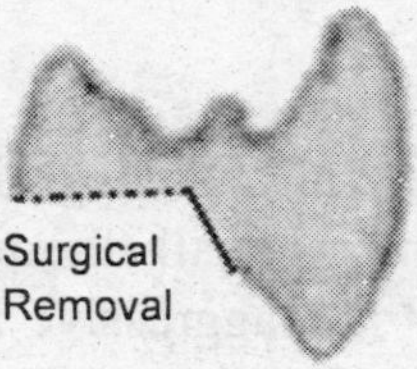

Partial Thyroid Lobectomy

This operation is not performed very often because there are not many conditions which will allow this limited approach. Additionally, a benign lesion must be ideally located in the upper or lower portion of one lobe for this operation to be a choice.

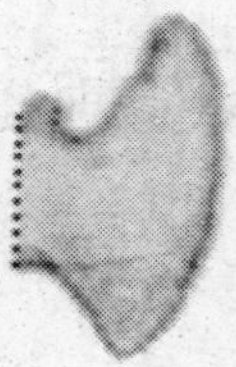

Thyroid Lobectomy

This is typically the "smallest" operation performed on the thyroid gland. It is performed for solitary dominant nodules which are worrisome for cancer or those which are indeterminate following fine needle biopsy. Also appropriate for follicular adenomas, solitary hot or cold nodules, or goiters which are isolated to one lobe (not common).

Thyroid Lobectomy with Isthmusectomy

This simply means removal of a thyroid lobe and the isthmus (the part that connects the two lobes). This removes more thyroid tissue than a simple lobectomy, and is used when a larger margin of tissue is needed to assure that the "problem" has been removed. Appropriate for those indications listed under thyroid lobectomy as well as for Hurthle cell tumors, and some very small and non-aggressive thyroid cancers.

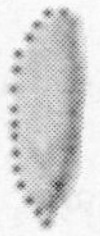

Subtotal Thyroidectomy

Just as the name implies, this operation removes all the "problem" side of the gland as well as the isthmus and the majority of the opposite lobe. This operation is typical for small, non-aggressive thyroid cancers. Also a common operation for goiters which are causing problems in the neck or even those which extend into the chest

Total Thyroidectomy

This operation is designed to remove all of the thyroid gland. It is the operation of choice for all thyroid cancers which are not small and non-aggressive in young patients. Many surgeons prefer this complete removal of thyroid tissue for **all** thyroid cancers regardless of the type

GOITRE

A goitre is a non-specific term that is used to describe any enlargement of the thyroid.

It is seen as a midline neck swelling which moves up on swallowing.

Goitres are more common in women than men.

Patterns of Thyroid Enlargement

Three patterns of thyroid enlargement are recognised:

- Diffuse:
  - painless:
  - iodine deficiency
  - simple goitre
  - goitrogens
  - dyshormogenesis
  - Grave's disease in remission
  - thyroiditis
  - infiltration, e.g. sarcoidosis
- Painful:
  - de Quervain's thyroiditis
  - Hashimoto's thyroiditis—rarely
- Multinodular
- Single nodule:
  - adenoma
  - carcinoma

Aetiology

Causes of goitre include:

- Physiological:
  - puberty—increased metabolic demand
  - pregnancy—increased demand; increased TBG
  - physiologic stress of any kind
- Autoimmune:
  - Graves' disease
  - Hashimoto's thyroiditis
- Thyroiditis:
  - subacute granulomatous/de Quervain's
  - subacute lymphocytic/silent
  - Riedel's thyroiditis—uncommon; gland usually shrinks
  - acute infective—transient
  - infiltrative e.g. sarcoidosis, tuberculosis
- Iodine deficiency—simple, endemic goitre

- idiopathic—simple, sporadic goitre
- Multinodular goitre—develops from simple goitre
- dyshormogenesis—including Pendred's syndrome:
  - Inability to use trapped iodine
  - Deficiency of peroxidase and dehalogenase
  - Abnormal protein binding in the plasma
- goitrogens
- thyroid cysts—rare
- thyroid tumour

History and Presentation

Many patients are asymptomatic. Features however, may include:

- pain—in association with:
  - Haemorrhage into a nodule
  - de Quervain's or rarely, Hashimoto's thyroiditis
  - Rapidly growing neoplasm
- Choking attacks—which may occur even with quite small goitres

Large, retrosternal tumours may cause:

- Obstruction of the great veins
- Dysphagia
- Stridor—if more than 75% of the diameter of the trachea is compressed

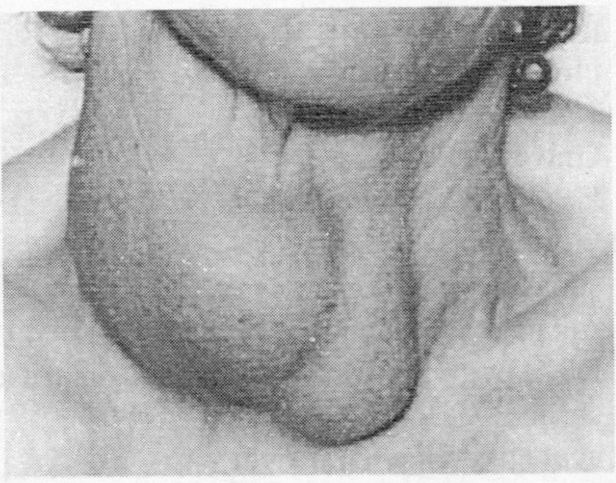

Fig. 4.6: Goitre

- Recurrent laryngeal palsy—rare

Examination may reveal a bruit, especially in a toxic goitre

Investigations

Assessment of thyroid physiology:

- Thyroid function tests—TSH, T4 or T3; mandatory in all patients with goitre

Assessment of thyroid morphology:

- Chest X-ray—detection of tracheal compression
- Chest CT—if suspect malignant change in a retrosternal thyroid
- Ultrasound scan—differentiates solid, partly cystic and cystic changes

Assessment of thyroid pathology:

- Isotope scan—now technetium rather than radio-iodine.
- Fine needle aspiration biopsy: ultrasonographically-guided biopsy is both highly sensitive and specific for pathology when compared with definitive diagnosis at post-operative pathological examination

Management

Diffuse, non-toxic goitre—small goitres usually require little treatment apart from reassurance and possibly iodine supplements. Large goitres may be treated by subtotal thyroidectomy since thyroxine causes shrinkage in less than 30% of cases.

The treatment of choice for thyrotoxicosis caused by thyroid nodular disease is radio-iodine (2).

Multinodular goitre—thyroxine is often successful in preventing progression and occasionally, in causing regression. **Surgery is indicated** if:

- There is retrosternal extension
- There is dysphagia attributed to the goitre
- There is marked tracheal deviation or stenosis

- There is a recurrent laryngeal palsy
- The goitre is cosmetically unacceptable
- The patient is hyperthyroid

A total thyroidectomy with lifelong thyroxine may be indicated if there is no normal thyroid tissue.

Solitary "cold" nodules"may be removed for cosmetic reasons or if shown to be malignant.

Solitary "hot" nodules—excised if associated with hyperthyroidism.

HYPOTHYROIDISM

Hypothyroidism describes the clinical syndrome which results from a deficiency of circulating thyroid hormones; myxoedema is a severe form of this syndrome and usually applied to cases in which deposition of mucinous substances results in thickening of the skin and subcutaneous tissues.

The prevalence is approximately 15 per 1000 in females and 1 per 1000 in males with a peak in the fifth or sixth decades. However, any age group may be affected.

Onset is extremely insidious and symptoms may be unnoticed for several years. Lethargy, fatigue and physical and mental slowness are common presenting features in adults; in children, cretinism may result.

Types

1. Congenital
2. Neonatal
3. Subclinical

Congenital hypothyroidism

Congenital hypothyroidism occurs in about 1 in 4000 live births in the UK, twice as often in females than in males.

The development of the central nervous system is intrinsically reliant on thyroxine from early foetal life, and some infants may have developed irreversible brain damage before birth. However, neonatal screening with the commencement of thyroxine therapy within 2 weeks of birth has enabled many infants to attain normal intellectual development.

Infants with primary hypothyroidism have raised TSH and lowered thyroxine.

Presenting features include:

- Coarse facies, with macroglossia
- Dry skin
- Hoarse cry
- Hypotonia
- Hypothermia
- Umbilical hernia
- **Prolonged jaundice**
- Constipation
- Presence of a goitre suggests a goitrogen aetiology
- The **posterior fontanelle remains open**, and closure of the anterior fontanelle is delayed
- The infant may be **anaemic**
- If untreated mental retardation may develop.

Treatment

This is by replacement with thyroxine, at first 25 micrograms per kilogram per day. The risk of over-treatment is advancement of bone age and subsequent reduced adult height; monitoring is therefore with growth measurement, bone age assessment and levels of free T4 and TSH.

With a stable clinical scenario children might require monitoring every few months in the first couple of years of life, falling to yearly monitoring after the 3rd birthday.

With such an apparently well child it is sometimes difficult for parents to remember to give thyroxine daily, but their memory may improve near to a clinic visit, relected by a normal T4 but a high TSH; the latter reflects a longer time period since it takes a longer time to correct.

Screening for congenital hypothyroidism : involves looking for high concentrations of neonatal blood TSH—this test discriminates better than low blood thyroxine, although it accepts a failure to recognise congenital pituitary hypothyroidism.

The screening works in parallel to the PKU screening program, so allowing it to be implemented at minimal extra cost and organisation.

The prevalence of this condition appears to have increased since the introduction of the program, and it is hard to decide if this is a true increase in prevalence or a reflection of overdiagnosis or previous underdiagnosis.

The test is repeated in those being treated with a withdrawal of the treatment at one year.

Neonatal Hypothyroidism

Hypothyroidism late in foetal life—for example from maternal iodine deficiency late in pregnancy—or during infancy affects somatic rather than neurological development. The hallmark of so called myxoedematous cretinism is marked growth retardation; intellectual development may not be impaired as thyroxine levels in the early critical phases of brain development are normal.

Diagnosis of neonatal hypothyroidism is readily confirmed by thyroid function tests and the condition responds well to thyroxine or iodine supplementation.

Subclinical Hypothyroidism

This is defined as an elevated serum TSH but a normal serum thyroxine concentration in an asymptomatic patient. The most common cause is chronic autoimmune thyroiditis (occurs in 3% of adults and 10% of postmenopausal women). Some patients with subclinical hypothyroidism will have common and nonspecific symptoms such as tiredness or weight gain.

The rate of progression from subclinical to overt hypothyroidism has been stated as less than 3% per annum (1). However, in those patients with positive thyroid antibodies, it can be that up to 80% of patients will develop overt hypothyroidism over a four year period (2).

Management

- Some authorities suggest it is better to treat subclinical hypothyroidism before overt hypothyroidism develops, especially in patients with positive thyroid antibodies as the rate of progression to overt hypothyroidism is much higher in these patients.
- In patients with only slightly raised TSH (less than 10 mU/L), without antithyroid antibodies (thyroid peroxidase autoantibodies), treatment may be deferred as the conversion rate to overt hypothyroidism is less than 3% per year (1).
- Increased TSH may be transient and may reflect a non-thyroidal illness or transient thyroiditis from which the patient is recovering.
  - do not start treatment on the basis of a single raised TSH level in people who are antibody negative (1,3)—it is prudent to repeat the measurement after about 3 months (2,3).
- Prodigy guidance suggests treatment should usually be commenced if diagnosis is confirmed on repeat testing 3 months later (3).
  - however if the TSH level is only slightly raised (less than 10 mU/l), and antithyroid antibodies are not present, then treatment may be deferred (providing follow-up is assured) (3).
- The aims of treatment is to restore serum TSH concentration to within the reference range; levels below this range may be associated with an increased risk of developing atrial fibrillation. However overall, the risks of thyroxine therapy are probably minimal provided the TSH is kept within the normal range, and a trial of treatment in symptomatic patients with subclinical hypothyroidism may be acceptable (2).

- if thyroxine therapy is initiated then a usual starting dose would be 50-100 mcg per day (although 25 mcg per day may be sufficient).
- start with 25 mcg daily and increase cautiously if coexistent heart disease or the elderly (3).

Aetiology

Hypothyroidism may be classified into:

- primary hypothyroidism where the pathology affect the thyroid gland itself.
- secondary hypothyroidism where the thyroid gland is normal but the production of stimulatory factors is disordered.

Investigations in hypothyroidism

- Primary hypothyroidism is indicated by a reduction in free and total T4, and elevated serum TSH.
- Elevated serum TSH with normal serum T4 indicates subclinical hypothyroidism.
- Free or total serum T3 is generally unhelpful since it may be only slightly reduced in severe hypothyroidism, or may be elevated by illness unrelated to thyroid function, or as a consequence of incorrect drug therapy.
- Secondary hypothyroidism is suggested by reduced free or total T4 and TSH below or within normal range; other tests for hypothalamic/ pituitary function are necessary.
- Other tests of thyroid function—e.g. thyroidal uptake tests, serum cholesterol have limited value in the diagnosis.
- Primary myxoedema may demonstrate a normal or exaggerated response of TSH to TRH; a negative TSH response excludes primary hypothyroidism but not a secondary cause.
- Antithyroid antibodies are suggestive of aetiology only.

Other possible features:

- Normochromic macrocytic anaemia.

- CK, AST and LDH may be elevated (due to abnormal muscle membranes).

Treatment of Hypothyroidism

Symptomatic patients are treated with thyroxine. Initially a relatively small dose of thyroxine (25—50 microgrammes per day) is given for the first four weeks and then this is altered depending on response. Normally, a single oral dose of 50-150 microgrammes per day is effective long term treatment.

Special consideration should be given to patients with ischaemic heart disease because the resultant increase in heart rate may precipitate worsening angina, myocardial infarction or even death. Thyroxine should be given in low dose—25 microgrammes daily or on alternate days—and in conjunction with beta blockers e.g. propranolol.

Dosage is increased gradually until euthyroidism is reached. Note that the half-life of thyroxine is approximately 7 days and therefore any change in dosage will take approximately 4 weeks to be assessed accurately by TSH test (TSH had a half-life on approximately 1 hour).

THYROIDITIS

The most common and well characterised forms of thyroiditis are:

- Hashimoto's or autoimmune thyroiditis
- De Quervains or subacute granulomatous thyroiditis
- subacute lymphocytic or painless thyroiditis
- Riedel's thyroiditis

Less common and less characterised forms are:

- Acute or infective thyroiditis
- Infiltrative thyroiditis e.g. sarcoidosis, tuberculosis.

Hashimoto's Thyroiditis

This is an autoimmune disorder characterised by extensive infiltration of the thyroid parenchyma by lymphocytes and plasma cells, with the formation of germinal centres. It is the most common cause of sporadic goitrous hypothyroidism in non-iodine deficient areas. Peak incidence is between 30 and 50 years of age with a female predominance of 15:1.

Pathogenesis

The basic defect in Hashimoto's disease appears to be a deficiency of antigen-specific suppressor T cells. This permits uncontrolled attack on the follicular cells by cytotoxic T cells with simultaneous unregulated T helper cell participation in the formation of auto-antibodies by B-cells.

The autoantibodies most consistently found in Hashimoto's disease are to the TSH receptor and to thyroid microsomes. Those to the TSH receptor are thyroid growth stimulating immunoglobulins. Less commonly, there are autoantibodies to thyroglobulin and to follicular cell membranes.

Thyroid enlargement probably reflects:

- Thyroid growth without increased hormone synthesis.
- Lymphocytic infiltration.
- Occasionally, increased TSH levels.

The thyroglobulin and thyroid microsomal antibodies are probably secondary to follicular cell damage initiated by cytotoxic T cells.

The association with the HLA-DR5 genotype may indicate a genetic predisposition to this pattern of autoantibody production.

It is associated with the HLA-DR5 genotype.

Morphology

Classically, the gland is symmetrically enlarged with the capsule intact and rarely adherent to the surrounding structures. Microscopically, there is extensive replacement of the gland by lymphocytes, plasma cells and macrophages with the formation of lymphoid germinal centres. Fibrosis is rare and confined to the interlobula septa.

The less common fibrosing variant shows less thyroid enlargement, less lymphoid infiltration and more fibrosis. Unlike Riedel's thyroiditis, however, the fibrosis does not extend beyond the capsule.

Clinical Features

Classically, presentation is with a goitre or hypothyroidism or both.

The thyroid may be barely palpable or greatly enlarged. Characteristically, it is firm, and well defined with an enlarged pyramidal lobe and palpable neighbouring lymph nodes. Enlargement is usually slow and painless but rarely, may be more rapid and painful.

At presentation, 75% of patients are euthyroid, 20% are hypothyroid, and 5% are hyperthyroid—a disease known as hashitoxicosis. About 50% eventually become hypothyroid because of destruction of the thyroid gland.

There appears to be an increased incidence of lymphoma but not of thyroid carcinoma.

Associated Conditions

Other autoimmune disorders associated with the disease include:

- Systemic lupus erythematous
- Rheumatoid arthritis
- Pernicious anaemia
- Vitiligo
- Type II diabetes mellitus
- Grave's disease
- Turner's syndrome—females with Turner's syndrome have a much higher incidence of autoimmune thyroiditis than the general population.

Diagnosis

The condition may be suspected clinically on the basis of the goitre with or without hypothyroidism.

Serum TSH is usually raised.

Measurement of antithyroid antibodies reveal:

- Antithyroid peroxidase antibodies (previously known as thyroid microsomal antibodies)—high titre.
- Thyroglobulin antibodies—low titre.

The gland may feel lumpy or irregular and biopsy may be necessary to distinguish it from a carcinoma of the thyroid. Surgical incision has been likened to cutting through an unripe pear.

If the patient is hypothyroid then oral thyroxine may keep the patient euthyroid and lead to resolution of the goitre.

de Quervain's thyroiditis

This is a distinctive form of self-limited thyroiditis noted for painful enlargement of the thyroid gland in association with fever and hyperthyroidism. It most commonly affects people in the second to fifth decade, with a female predominance of 3:1. The condition is widely believed to be triggered by a virus infection—mumps, influenza, Coxsackie, adenovirus or ECHO.

Characteristically, levels of T3 and T4 are increased but the uptake of radioactive iodine is low or absent.

Pathophysiology

The early stages are characterised by glandular enlargement, follicular disruption and neutrophilic invasion. Later, macrophages and multinucleate giant cells are seen enveloping fragments of colloid. These resemble granulomas.

Viral antibodies are detectable in about half of cases.

The initial transient hyperthyroidism is produced by the leakage of preformed thyroid hormones from the damaged follicular cells. Follicular disruption also explains the low or absent uptake of radioactive iodine.

The ensuing transient hypothyroidism is due to gland destruction. Regeneration of the follicles, usually from the edges of the most severely affected areas, results in restoration of thyroid function.

Clinical Features

Presentation is with:

- Sudden, painful enlargement of the thyroid mimicking a "sore throat" or "ear ache"
- Flu-like symptoms
- General features of hyperthyroidism

Typically, both lobes are enlarged but rarely, one lobe is affected. Painful dysphagia is common.

Blood tests reveal high ESR, raised T4 and T3, and suppressed TSH. Uptake of radioactive iodine is low.

Characteristically, the condition progresses through a phase of transient hyperthyroidism, followed 4-6 weeks later by a similar period of transient hypothyroidism. The patient is usually euthyroid 4-6 months after the onset of the illness.

Management

- Beta blockers may be required to control toxic symptoms in the hyperthyroid phase.
- Pain in the thyroid usually responds to aspirin but in more severe cases, may require a short course of prednisolone.

Relapses occur in up to 47% of patients, usually in the first year.

Subacute Lymphocytic Thyroiditis

- Subacute lymphocytic thyroiditis may present with painless goitrous enlargement or hyperthyroidism, or both. Generally, the levels of T3 and T4 are raised, while thyroid uptake of radioactive iodine is low.
- The condition is relatively common in the USA where it may account for 15% of all cases of

hyperthyroidism. It is less common in the UK. Silent thyroiditis may occur at any age but is most frequently reported in the 12 months following childbirth—so called post-partum thyroiditis.

- Aetiology is obscure. There is no clear association with viral infection, de Quervains thyroiditis, Hashimoto's disease or primary hypothyroidism. This condition is mediated by antithyroid peroxidase antibodies (formerly known as antimicrosomal antibodies) and thyroid stimulating immunoglobulin (as seen in Graves' disease) are not present (1).
- Morphologically, it is characterised by foci of lymphocytic infiltration, sometimes with increased interstitial fibrous tissue. There are no lymphoid germinal centres and few, if any, plasma cells
- The condition is self-limiting. Hyperthyroidism is commonly followed by a phase of hypothyroidism may become permanent in 25% of patients (1).
- Patients with this condition are referred for pecialist management.
- Antithyroid drugs and radioiodine are unhelpful—this is because hyperthyroidism is secondary to thyroid distruction causing increased thyroxine release. Beta blockers may provide symptomatic relief.

Riedel's Thyroiditis

This is an extremely rare sclerosing disease of unknown aetiology. It is characterised by replacement of the thyroid parenchyma with dense fibrous tissue which extends beyond the thyroid capsule into surrounding structures in the neck. Peak incidence is in the fourth to seventh decade with a female predominance of 3:1.

Usually, the main complaint is of a painless lump in the neck. Rarely, there may be dysphagia, dyspnoea, stridor, or suffocation. Hypothyroidism occurs in 25-50% of cases. The thyroid is woody or iron-hard. It is usually markedly contracted and difficult to palpate. Rarely, it may be of normal size or slightly enlarged. Occasionally there may be features of compression.

The condition may resemble an infiltrating carcinoma and may be associated with other idiopathic fibrosing conditions such as sclerosing cholangitis and fibrous mediastinitis.

Surgery may be needed to relieve pressure on the trachea. It is uncommon for thyroidectomy to be required.

Thyroiditis (acute)

Infection of the thyroid is rare. It usually occurs in young children or debilitated patients. Most often, it occurs secondary to infection elsewhere.

Bacterial infection is most common. Agents include staphylococcal aureus—in one third of cases—streptococci, Salmonella, Enterobacter and mycobacteria. Fungal infection is rare.

Presentation is usually with painful enlargement of the thyroid gland.

The condition is usually transient. It may be treated with surgical drainage and antibiotics.

Long term thyroid dysfunction is rare.

Chapter 5

Adrenal Gland Diseases

PHAEOCHROMOCYTOMA

Phaeochromocytomas are functional tumours that arise from chromaffin cells in the adrenal medulla. They account for 0.1-0.2% of cases of systemic hypertension.

Phaeochromocytomas usually secrete a combination of noradrenaline and adrenaline, but some tumours may also secrete dopamine and rarely ACTH causing Cushing's syndrome.

Neoplasms of chromaffin cells may also arise in other parts of the body. By convention those arising outside the adrenal gland are referred to as extra-adrenal paragangliomas. Of these, chromaffin tumours arising from aorticosympathetic paraganglia have histologic, biochemical and clinical similarities to phaeochromocytomas and are sometimes referred to as extra-adrenal phaeochromocytomas.

TEN PERCENT RULE

Phaeochromocytomas may be referred to as the 10% tumour:

- 10% are extra-adrenal, most commonly, in the organ of Zuckerkandl, located in the aortic bifurcation. Less than 1% are extra-abdominal.
- 10% are bilateral, increasing to 70% in familial cases.
- 10% are malignant, but the risk of malignancy in women is three fold that in men.
- 10% are multiple.

- 10% occur in children, but 25-30% of children have extra-adrenal and/or bilateral tumors.

Aetiology

The aetiology is not known but a significant genetic component is recognised. Ten percent are familial. These are invariably adrenal in origin, and are bilateral in 70%.

Phaechromocytomas may be associated with:

- Multiple endocrine neoplasia—MEN IIa, MEN IIb
- Other neuroectodermal disease:
  - neurofibromatosis—in 5% of cases of phaeochromocytoma.
  - von Hippel Lindau syndrome—rarely.
  - tuberous sclerosis.

Tumours that arise in association with MEN-II or von Hippel Lindau syndrome, in general, affect younger age groups.

Pathology

Phaeochromocytomas may arise as one or more discrete neoplasms within the adrenal medulla and particularly in MEN syndromes there may be surrounding diffuse or nodular hyperplasia.

The tumour mass varies widely but on average is approximately 100 gms. Large tumours may be encapsulated by connective tissue, and may contain areas of haemorrhage, necrosis or cyst formation. The cut surface may be grey or brown in colour, and the tumour due to its stored catecholamines reacts histochemically to dichromate producing a brown-black colouring.

Tumour cells resemble those of the normal adrenal medulla by being arranged in nests. There may be mitotic figures or nuclear pleomorphism, and tumour cells may be found in capillaries or sinusoids. None of these features however indicate that the tumour is one of the ten percent of phaeochromocytomas that are malignant. Malignancy may only be proved by the finding of distal metastases.

Clinical Features

All ages and races can be affected. The peak incidence is in the third and fourth decades of life. Men and women are equally affected.

Hypertension is the usual presenting feature. This may be sustained or paroxysmal with intervening periods of normotension.

Other symptoms related to catecholamine excess may present acutely as a hypertensive crisis, with features such as:

- Headache
- Palpitations
- Tachycardia
- Sweating
- Anxiety
- Panic attacks
- Tremor
- Nausea and vomiting
- Fever.

Virtually any stress can precipitate an attack, for example, exercise, emotion, postural changes, diagnostic procedures, or surgery. Occasionally, attacks occur spontaneously. Rarely, they are fatal.

Patients may show typical cardiovascular, cerebrovascular, and renal effects of prolonged hypertension, such as congestive heart failure with pulmonary oedema.

The diagnosis of phaeochromocytoma should be suspected:

- In any hypertensive with orthostatic hypotension and tachycardia.
- In any hypertensive whose symptoms respond poorly to anti-hypertensive treatment.
- In any patient whose blood pressure fluctuates widely.
- In any hypertensive with cafe au lait spots.

Diagnosis

A diagnosis of phaeochromocytoma can be confirmed from:

- 24 hour urinary free catecholamines, VMA's
- High performance liquid chromatography assay of plasma adrenaline and noradrenaline. Samples must be taken from an indwelling catheter to avoid the consequences of stress at the time of venepuncture. However, this is said to be the most reliable method of diagnosis.
- Clonidine suppression test
- pentolinium suppression test.

The tumour may be localised by:

- Abdominal CT
- MIBG scanning
- Adrenal angiography.

Differential Diagnosis

Phaeochromocytoma is a great mimic. Its differential diagnosis includes:

- Essential hypertension
- Migraine
- Thyrotoxicosis
- Alcohol withdrawal
- Carcinoid syndrome
- Hypoglycaemia
- Angina pectoris
- Pre-eclampsia, eclampsia or simple hypertension of pregnancy.

Management

Initial pharmacological treatment permits optimal surgical interventions. Alpha adrenoreceptor blockade with phenoxybenzamine is commenced a few days before beta blockade with propranolol. The intravascular hypovolaemia is corrected over 7-10 days prior to surgery.

The tumour is localised using the following imaging methods:

- CT scan—which can detect tumours greater than 1 cm in diameter.
- 131 I-meta-iodobenzylguanidine (MIBG) scintigraphy:
  - more sensitive than CT
  - MIBG is specifically concentrated in adrenergic cells and is useful for assessing metastases.

Surgery is curative in 75% of cases.

Excessive handling of the tumour peroperatively should be avoided as this may release large amounts of catecholamine into the circulation resulting in severe, acute hypertension.

Vasodilators such as sodium nitroprusside, and intra-venous alpha- and beta-blockers should be available during surgery in the event of a hypertensive crisis.

Operative mortality is at least 3%.

When surgery is not possible, consider treatment with:

- Phenoxybenzamine and propranolol
- Alpha-methyl-p-tyrosine—inhibits the hydroxylation of tyrosine to dopa and so, reduces synthesis of adrenaline and noradrenaline.

Prognosis

Prognosis is dependent on the presence or absence of complications of hypertension e.g. cerebrovascular accident, renal impairment.

- Mortality from elective surgery—less than 2%; approximately 80% of patients become normotensive following surgery.
- Ninety six percent 5-year survival with benign disease.
- Forty five percent 5-year survival with malignant disease.
- Recurrence rate—less than 10%.

ADRENOCORTICAL TUMOURS

Adrenocortical tumours account for about 25% of the cases of hypercortisolism. About 50% of adrenocortical tumours are malignant.

Clinical features

Adrenocortical tumours may cause:
- Hypercortisolism
- Virilising or feminising syndromes, including pseudoprecocious puberty
- They can also be a cause of hyperaldosteronism.

Treatment of Adrenocortical Tumours

Treatment is by surgical excision.

Treatment of recurrent tumours can be achieved by drug therapy, for example metyrapone for Cushing's syndrome due to adrenal adenoma, op'-DDD used for treatment of Cushing's syndrome due to adrenal carcinoma. Patients with Conn's syndrome which is the result of an inoperable tumour may be treated with spironolactone—an aldosterone antagonist.

Chapter 6

Breast Diseases and Conditions

- Congenital abnormalities and disorders of development and involution
- Breast infection
- Breast trauma
- Neoplastic
- Gynaecomastia.

Breast Problems: Congenital, Developmental and Involutional

Congenital:

- Extra nipples and breasts
- Absence/hypoplasia of the breast.

Aberrations of breast development:

- Juvenile or virginal hypertrophy
- Fibroadenomas.

Aberrations of involution:

- fibroadenosis
  - cystic disease
  - sclerosis
- duct ectasia
- galactocoele
- epithelial hyperplasia.

congenital Breast Abnormalities

The breasts are identical in boys and girls until puberty. Growth of the breast then begins in girls at about the age of 10. This growth may begin asymmetrically and may appear to be a breast lump. It should however not be biopsied as there is a risk of damaging the breast bud.

Accessory Nipples and Breasts

These may affect 1-5% of men and women, and they occur along the milk lines running from each axilla to the groin. Accessory nipples most commonly occur below the normal breast, whilst accessory breast tissue most commonly occurs in the lower axilla.

Treatment may be required for cosmetic reasons.

Nipple Disorders

Nipple disorders include:

- Inversion
- Eczema
- Discharge.

Nipple Inversion

Nipple inversion can be caused by:

- Congenital deformation
- Carcinoma
- Mammary duct ectasia with periductal fibrosis.

Nipple Eczema

Nipple eczema may be caused by:

- Paget's disease of the nipple
- Eczema.

Nipple Discharge

Nipple discharge can be of varied form:

- Clear—physiological
- Milky:
  - pregnancy—normal lactation
  - hyperprolactinaemia resulting in galactorrhoea.
- Brown or green:
  - perimenopausal
  - mammary duct ectasia
  - fibroadenosis.

- bloodstained:
  - carcinoma
  - intraductal papilloma.

Aberrations of Breast Development

Breasts develop throughout puberty and then continue to undergo cyclical changes with the menstrual cycle. In the event of pregnancy the breasts double their weight at term.

Many benign conditions in the developing and mature phases of the life cycle of the breast occur so often that they might be considered to be aberrations rather than disease.

Juvenile Breast Hypertrophy

This commonly presents in women under 25 whose breasts have grown normally throughout puberty but then continue to grow.

Their large breasts may cause them embarrassment, pain, discomfort and prevent them from performing everyday tasks.

No endocrine abnormality can be detected in these patients and treatment is with reduction mammoplasty, often resulting in a much improved quality of life.

Fibroadenoma of the Breast

While often considered a benign neoplasm, fibroadenomas may be thought of as aberrations of normal development. Unlike neoplasms breast fibroadenomas develop from a whole lobule rather than a single cell, and like normal breast tissue they remain responsive to hormonal control. Fibroadenomas are composed of both fibrous and glandular tissue.

Fibroadenomas are common and account for 13% of all symptomatic breast lumps. They are most common in women in their second or third decade, accounting for 60% of breast lumps in this younger population.

The tumour is well demarcated from the surrounding breast tissue by a condensed connective tissue capsule.

The tumour develops from a whole lobule and not from a single cell. Microscopically, the tumour comprises proliferation of the connective tissue stroma and atypical multiplication of ducts and acini.

Two histological patterns are noted:

- Pericanicular—connective tissue stroma surrounds small islands of glandular tissue, in a whorled pattern.
- Intracanicular—connective tissue stroma predominates and compresses the gland spaces; the epithelial elements appear as narrow strands or cords of epithelium lying within the fibrous tissue.

Clinical Features and Diagnosis

Presentation is usually as a discrete, firm, non-tender and highly mobile nodule within the breast. Small lesions may slip away from the examining hand during palpation giving rise to their description as "breast mice." A few patients may present with multiple fibroadenomas.

Diagnosis may be made with a combination of clinical assessment, ultrasonography and fine needle aspiration cytology. Fibroadenomas in older patients may calcify and give characteristic mammographic appearances.

Management

Less than 5% of fibroadenomas increase in size and about 25% either get smaller or completely disappear.

The difficulty in management however is to ensure that breast cancer is not missed, and some would advocate that all such lumps should be excised, thus providing both diagnosis and treatment.

Others however would argue that for women under 40 years old, with a fibroadenoma diagnosed clinically, with ultrasound and with fine needle aspiration cytology, excision is not required unless the lump is over 4 cms in diameter. For women over 40 years old, all lumps should be excised.

Fibrocystic Disease of Breast

Fibroadenosis or fibrocystic disease is the most common cause of breast lumps in women of reproductive age. The peak incidence is between 35 and 50 years of age. It is rare before 25 years.

The term embraces a spectrum of histologic changes, and may encompass many patients who have cystic lesions detected clinically or sclerotic breast lesions detected on mammography as discussed elsewhere.

Histologically it is characterized by overgrowth of both fibrous stroma, and of epithelial elements i.e. ducts and lobules, in differing proportions. These changes may be considered as abberations of normal breast involution and not part of a disease process. The condition may be due to a disordered or imbalanced response to endogenous sex hormones.

Only in those cases showing marked epithelial hyperplasia—epitheliosis—is the risk of breast carcinoma thought to be increased.

Pathology

A variety of changes may be noted including:

- Cysts:
  - microcysts—less than 1 cm in diameter
  - macrocysts—up to 5 cm in diameter; includes the blue domed cysts of Bloodgood which unopened, appear brown to blue due to the contained fluid.
- Apocrine metaplasia—the normal ductular epithelium that lines the cyst proliferates to resemble that of apocrine sweat glands.
- Fibrosis—proliferation of fibrous tissue without epithelial change.

- adenosis:
  - simple adenosis—hyperplastic proliferation of lobular acini/ductules.
  - sclerosing adenosis—proliferation of fibrous tissue accompanies that of the acini, splitting them apart.

Clinical Features

Typically, patients present with one or more lumps in the breast which may be painful, and frequently, bilateral. The size and pain usually vary with the menstrual cycle. One or more of these elements may be absent.

Cysts are more common in perimenopausal women. They are usually single. The presence of multiple, diffuse cysts may be referred to as Schimmelbusch's disease. The discharge varies from clear to green but should not be bloodstained.

On palpation, a cyst may be recognised by its smooth texture and characteristic tense fluctuation.

Management

Carcinoma must be excluded.

A discrete lump thought clinically to be a cyst should be aspirated. The lesion is benign if:

- The fluid is not bloodstained
- The lump completely disappears
- The cyst does not refill
- Cytology is negative.

If the lump is solid, or one of the above conditions is not upheld, mammography or preferably, excision biopsy is indicated.

Pain that is localised, is normally relieved by excision. Pain that is diffuse, cannot be relieved by excision. In these cases, bromocriptine, or danazol, may be helpful.

Aberrations of Involution

After pregnancy or in nulliparous women after the age of 30, the breast begins to involute.

During this process the breast stroma—the fibrous connective tissue which supports the glandular tissue of the breast—is gradually replaced by fat. This results in the breasts becoming less radiodense, softer and allowing them to droop. The glandular elements of the breast also change with areas of fibrosis, the formation of small cysts and an increase in the number of glandular elements or adenosis.

Duct ectasia (mammary)

Mammary duct ectasia refers to dilatation of the large and intermediate breast ducts. It results from the shortening and dilation of subareola ducts as they involute. In a small proportion of individuals excessively dilated ducts may present with a breast lump or nipple discharge.

Clinical Features

Patients are most commonly in the decade around the menopause or older. It has been estimated that by the age of 70, 40% of women have a substantial degree of duct ectasia.

Presentation is usually with a hard or doughy tender lump beneath or close to the areola, and nipple discharge which is often cheesy but may be green or blood stained. There may be slit-like nipple retraction.

The condition may be complicated by secondary infection.

Dilated ducts may be seen on mammography.

Differentiation from carcinoma may be difficult clinically.

Management

Surgery may be required to exclude malignancy, if the discharge is troublesome or to evert the nipple. Sub-areolar excision of all the major ducts may be necessary if the ectasia is extensive.

Galactocoele

A galactocoele is a cystic lesion of the breast which occurs after the cessation of lactation. It is due to obstruction of a lactiferous duct which becomes distended with milk and epithelial cells.

Patients usually present with a subareolar mass and milky nipple discharge. Secondary infection may produce foci of acute mastitis or abscess formation.

Treatment is by excision.

Epithelial Hyperplasia (breast)

This condition is identified histologically by an increase in the number of cells lining the terminal duct lobular unit. Hyperplasia may be graded as mild, moderate or florid and there may be atypia.

The presence of atypia is associated with a significantly increased risk of subsequent breast carcinoma.

BREAST INFECTION

1. Lactating Breast Infection

Breast feeding may cause abrasion of the skin around the breast and, on occasion, cracking of the nipple. This permits the entry of infective organisms, most commonly Staphylococcus aureus but also Staphylococcus epidermidis and streptococci. This may result in a circumareolar breast abscess, or deep infection of the lactiferous ducts.

Uncommonly, infections arise in the sebaceous glands (of Montgomery) of the areola.

Clinical Features

The initial presentation is that of a diffuse cellulitis which localises into an abscess after several days.

The patient may be generally unwell with a spiking fever. The affected area of the breast is painful and tender, red and warm. There may be a purulent discharge if the lesion is extensive.

Management

Breast milk should be obtained for culture and sensitivity.

Blind therapy is with flucloxacillin, assuming infection with staphylococcus. Other antibiotics which may adversely effect the baby should of course be avoided. Use erythromycin if penicillin-allergic.

Continuing breast feeding should be encouraged as this helps to drain the affected segment of the breast. It is important to empty the affected breast and if it is too tender for feeding to continue, the baby should be fed from the non-infected breast and milk expressed from the infected one.

If the infection persists after an initial course of flucloxacillin (and results of culture and sensitivity are not available), then co-amoxiclav, which has a wider spectrum of action, may be tried.

Any abscess which develops should be recurrently aspirated or incised and drained.

If inflammation or an associated mass persists, the possibility of underlying breast carcinoma should be considered and investigated with further imaging or needle biopsy.

Non-lactating Breast Infection

Breast infection in non-lactating women most commonly occurs in the periareolar region of the breast. Less commonly however, in patients with certain pre-existing conditions such as diabetes, infection may also be seen in peripheral breast tissue.

A. Periareolar Non-lactating Breast Infection

This is a condition where non-dilated subareolar breasts ducts become infected. It most commonly affects young women, with a mean age of 32 years.

The condition may present with periareolar inflammation, and the breast may be tender. There may be a history of nipple discharge and on examination the nipple may be retracted and there may be an associated inflammatory mass or abscess.

As with other breast infections treatment is with appropriate antibiotics, and abscesses should be aspirated or incised and drained.Any residual inflammation or masses following treatment should be further investigated to exclude a neoplasm.Recurrent breast infection or abscesses require surgery to remove the diseased duct.A common complication of draining a periareolar abscess is the formation of a mammary duct fistula.

B. Peripheral Non-lactating Breast Infection

Infections affecting peripheral portions of the breast are uncommon, but when they occur they are often associated with a pre-existing condition such as diabetes, rheumatoid arthritis, steroid treatment and trauma. Infections may also occur as part of a condition known as granulomatous lobular mastitis.

Pilonidal abscesses may also affect the breasts, particularly in sheep shearers and hairdressers.

Infective organisms may be aerobic or anaerobic and include Staphylococcus aureus, Enterococci, Anaerobic streptococci and Bacteroides species.

As with other breast infections antibiotics should be prescribed, and if there are abscesses these should be recurrently aspirated or incised and drained.

3. Skin Associated Breast Infection

The skin of the breast may become affected by cellulitis or abscess formation following direct infection often by Staphylococcus aureus or rarely certain fungi.

Such infections occur in women whose skin has been damaged by previous surgery or radiotherapy, but also occur in women predisposed to infection due to being overweight, having large breasts or due to poor personal hygiene.Treatment is with appropriate antibiotics and the aspiration or incision and drainage of abscesses.

Advice may be given if necessary about weight loss, keeping the breasts as clean and dry as possible i.e. avoiding talc, skin creams and the wearing of a cotton bra or cotton T shirt under a bra.

In cases of hidradenitis suppurativa, excision of affected skin prevents further infection in a proportion of patients.

BREAST NEOPLASMS

Classification:

- Benign
- Pre-malignant
- Malignant:
  - primary:
    - § carcinoma in situ
    - § invasive breast carcinoma
  - secondary.

Benign Breast Tumours

Classification:

- Epithelial:
  - intraduct papilloma
  - adenoma i.e. an excess of ductules.
- Mesenchymal:
  - lipoma
  - fibroma.
- Mixed:
  - fibroadenomas
  - Phyllodes tumours.

Note fibroadenomas though included here are not true neoplasms. They originate from a whole group of cells and are so common that they are best considered as abberations of normal development rather than neoplastic in origin.

Intraductal Papilloma

Intraductal papillomas are localised areas of epithelial proliferation within large mammary or lactiferous ducts. The lesions may occur singly or as part of the multiple intraductal papillomatosis syndrome which has an increased risk of malignancy.

Patient's are generally premenopausal and present with nipple discharge and bleeding. A small, painful subareolar nodule is present in 30% of cases.

The condition must be distinguished from Paget's disease, adenoma of the nipple, and carcinoma. A mammogram is indicated. The injection of contrast—ductography—may identify the papilloma as a filling defect.

Treatment is by surgical excision of the affected segment of breast tissue—microdochectomy.

Phyllodes Tumours

Phyllodes tumours consist of mixed epithelial and connective tissue elements but have greater stromal cellularity than fibroadenomas.

Benign and malignant tumours are recognised. Distinction is made on cytological grounds such as cellular irregularity and mitotic activity. Most of the tumours previously termed cytosarcoma phyllodes fall into the benign group.

Phyllodes tumours usually develop in women over the age of 35 years but may occur in young girls around the menarche.

Presentation is usually with a bulky, lobulated mass which greatly enlarges and distorts the breast. The overlying skin is red and warm, reflecting the increased vascularity.

In large tumours, pressure skin necrosis may develop. In these, the capsule of the tumour may rupture, and the growth fungate through the skin as an irregular mass.

Management depends on the age of the patient. In those less than 20 years of age, malignant transformation is rare so that the condition may be regarded as benign. Simple enucleation through a submammary incision is sufficient.

Phyllodes tumours in older patients show a marked tendency to local recurrence. Treatment is by local excision with a good clearance. Mastectomy may be indicated for extensive lesions, older patients, or in patients with small breasts. Local treatment is identical for benign and malignant tumours.

The prognosis for benign phyllodes tumour after surgery is excellent. That for malignant phyllodes tumour depends on the size of the lesion and the histological findings. It is poor for tumours greater than 10 cm diameter and with more than ten mitoses per ten high power fields.

Breast Carcinoma in situ

In situ carcinoma of the breast is characterised by the proliferation of malignant epithelial cells within the ducts or lobules without invasion of the surrounding stroma. It represents the earliest stage of breast cancer, and probably, the best opportunity for cure.

Two patterns are defined:
- ductal carcinoma *in situ*
- lobular carcinoma *in situ*.

Ductal Carcinoma in Situ of Breast

In ductal carcinoma in situ, the malignant cells are epithelial, confined to the ducts and do not invade the basement membrane. It is associated with an increased risk of invasive breast carcinoma. The risk of invasive carcinoma is increased in proportion to the extent of in situ disease.

In the general population, the incidence of ductal carcinoma *in situ* is about 5%. However, in populations screened mammographically, this increases to 15-20% due to the tendency to produce conspicuous microcalcification. Most cases are detected by mammography whilst asymptomatic. Previously, diagnosis was made at a late stage when the lesion was palpable e.g. a firm mass or 'ropy' cords, or had caused other symptoms, as in Paget's disease. Usually, only one breast is affected.

The introduction of breast screening has seen a 3-4 fold increase in the diagnosis of DCIS.

Two broad types of ductal carcinoma in situ are recognised:

- Comedo-type tumours are characterised by:
  - pleomorphic cells ductal epithelial cells obliterate the lumina of the ducts and grow along them.
  - eventually solid cords of anaplastic cells
  - central necrosis
  - microcalcification
  - associated with multicentric disease
  - high expression of C-erb2 oncogene.
- Non-comedo type tumours are characterised by:
  - variable histology:
    - § cribriform
    - § micropapillary
    - § clinging
    - § solid.
  - less frequent:
  - mitoses
    - § necrosis
    - § calcification.

Often, comedo and non-comedo types occur simultaneously.

Management

Untreated, DCIS is associated with a substantially increased risk of developing invasive carcinoma:

- Comedo type—50% become invasive within 3 years.
- Non-comedo type—30% become invasive within 10-15 years.

The optimal therapy remains controversial but should involve local resection with pathologically clear margins. This may be combined with various combinations of radiotherapy and/or tamoxifen. Regular follow-up with clinical examination and mammography is advised.

For women with widespread or multifocal microcalcifications, with Paget's disease, or who are elderly, a simple mastectomy may be preferred.

Lobular Carcinoma *in Situ* of Breast

LCIS commonly occurs in premenopausal women. The incidence is unknown as there are no distinctive clinical or radiologic features. The condition is usually discovered as an incidental finding when a biopsy is made for otherwise benign disease. There are no clear mammographic features. Clinically, it is not palpable and does not tend to metastasize.

LCIS is frequently bilateral and multicentric. It is associated with an eleven-fold increased risk of subsequent invasive carcinoma. There is no relation between the breast in which LCIS is detected and that in which invasive carcinoma occurs. LCIS is regarded as a marker of increased risk anywhere in the breast. Thirty percent of patients develop invasive carcinoma within 15-20 years. This is a lower relative risk than ductal carcinoma *in situ*.

Management consists of lifelong surveillance by annual mammography and clinical examination. As the majority of patients are premenopausal, the use of Tamoxifen may alter the hormonal milieu and diminish the risk of invasive carcinoma.

BREAST CANCER

Breast cancer is the commonest malignancy in women, accounting for 20% of all cancer deaths in females.

One in eleven women will suffer from breast cancer. The annual age adjusted death rate is approximately 27 per 100,000.

These statistics and the accessibility of the breast to screening procedures have provided the impetus for national breast cancer screening programmes.

Risk Factors

The clearest risks for invasive breast cancer are:
- Female sex
- The presence of preinvasive cancer:
  - lobular carcinoma *in situ*
  - ductal carcinoma *in situ*.

- Previous breast cancer

Other risk factors (classified as increased risk above normal) include:

- family history of breast cancer—the risk of breast cancer in a woman has been quantified with respect to the number of affected first degree relatives and by the age of affected first degree relative (1).

Table 6.1: Relative risk for breast cancer by number of affected first degree female relatives

Number of first degree relatives	*Relative risk for women < 50 years (99% CI)*	*Relative risk for women >= 50 years (CI)*
1	2.14 (1.92 to 2.38)	1.65 (1.53 to 1.78)
2	3.84 (2.37 to 6.22)	2.61 (2.03 to 3.34)
3	12.05 (1.70 to 85.16)	2.65 (1.29 to 5.46)

Table 6.2: Relative risk for breast cancer by age of affected first degree relative

Age at time of diagnosis in first degree relatives	*Relative risk for women < 50 years (99% CI)*	*Relative risk for women >= 50 years (CI)*
< 40 years	13.5 (3.4 to 53.9)	3.9 (1.8 to 8.6)
>= 40 years	7.8 (2.4 to 25.0)	2.6 (1.8 to 3.7)

- Age—peak incidence 45-75 years but any age postmenarche >> 4x.
- Country of residence—high in West > 4x e.g. UK, low in East e.g. Japan
- Previous breast cancer > 4x.
- Irradiation of chest—shows a linear dose-response relationship 2-4x.
- Social class (I vs. V) 2-4x.
- Race—more common in Caucasians < 2x.
- Previous ovarian or endometrial cancer < 2x.
- Early menarche or late menopause < 2x.
- Nulliparity or older than 30 years before first child < 2x.
- Hormonal supplementation < 2x.
- Obesity—oestrogen synthesis in adipose tissue.
- Alcohol consumption.

In the male, Klinefelter's syndrome is a risk factor for breast cancer.

Histological Classification

- Carcinoma of no special type ("ductal") 60-70 %
- Carcinoma of special type:
  - Tubular 1-5 %
  - medullary < 5 %
  - mucinous < 5 %
  - papillary 1 %.
- Infiltrating lobular carcinoma 10-20% (may be bilateral).
- Mixed—ductal, lobular, rare types 10%.

Grading of a tumour is based on—degree of glandular formation, mitotic rate, nuclear pleomorphism; each scored from 1-3. Score.

- Well differentiated—grade I (3-5).
- Moderately differentiated—grade II (6-7).
- Poorly differentiated—grade III (8-9).

Clinical Presentation

Breast cancer may be asymptomatic, occurring as an impalpable lesion on screening mammogram. (Upto 70% of important mammographic lesions are impalpable).

In other cases, patients may present with:

- Palpable breast lump:
  - 40-50% in the upper outer quadrant
  - 70-80% scirrhous i.e. hard and encapsulated
  - may be tethered to superficial or deep structures
  - does not fluctuate or transilluminate
  - 15-40% multicentric
  - bilateral in up to 30% of cases of lobular carcinoma
  - frequently, patient detected.
- Skin changes:
  - dimpling
  - peau d'orange
  - nipple "eczema" in Paget's

- visible lump
- surface ulceration; neglected carcinoma in elderly.

- Recent nipple inversion.
- Bloodstained nipple discharge—uncommon.
- Non-cyclic breast pain—usually, a late sign.
- Disseminated disease:
  - Bone pain, pathological fracture
  - Dyspnoea, pleural effusion
  - Hepatomegaly, jaundice.

Diagnosis

The diagnosis of breast cancer must be made with certainty before surgery can be undertaken. The diagnosis cannot be made on history and examination alone.

Investigative measures to confirm the diagnosis include:

- Imaging:
  - mammography
  - ultrasound
  - ductography.
- Biopsy:
  - fine needle aspiration biopsy
  - core needle biopsy
  - localisation biopsy
  - open biopsy.
- Detection of metastatic disease:
  - liver function tests
  - serum calcium
  - chest radiograph
  - isotope bone scan
  - liver ultrasound scan
  - CT brain.

The yield from an extensive search for metastatic disease is poor except in cases where suspicion is great clinically. Hence, symptoms of metastasis or patients with stage III disease should have a bone scan, chest X ray and liver ultrasound. A CT scan of the brain should only be carried out when the history or examination is suggestive of metastasis e.g. fits.

TNM Staging of Breast Cancer

- T0—no evidence of primary tumour.
- T1—the tumour is 2 cm or less in diameter, with no skin involvement—except in the case of Paget's disease where confined to the nipple—and no nipple retraction or fixation.
- T2—tumour greater than 2 cm but less than 5 cm.
- T3—tumour greater than 5 cm in greatest diameter, less than 10 cm.
- T4—greater than 10 cm or skin or chest wall involvement or peau d'orange.
- N0—no palpable ipsilateral axillary nodes.
- N1—palpable, ipsilateral axillary nodes.
- N2—ipsilateral axillary nodal metastases fixed to one another or to other structures.
- N3—metastases to ipsilateral internal mammary nodes.
- M0—no evidence of metastases.
- M1—distant metastases (includes ipsilateral supraclavicular nodes).

Management of Breast Cancer

The management of breast cancer is determined by the stage of the disease and in part, the patient's wishes. Patient involvement has been shown to reduce the incidence of anxiety and depression after treatment.

Breast cancer management in recent years has moved away from radical to conservative surgery. This has occured due to a change in theory of how breast cancer disseminates—see submenu.

Management requires a multidisciplinary approach entailing input from:

- Surgeon
- Breast care nurse
- Pathologist e.g. FNAC at time of clinic
- Radiologist e.g. mammography
- Oncologist e.g. in advanced disease
- Psychiatrist e.g. in event of depressive illness
- Plastic surgeon e.g. for breast reconstruction.

Management may be considered to consist of a combination of:

- Local treatments to control local disease
- Systemic treatments to treat micrometastatic disease.

The aims of local management are to:

- Remove the local tumour reducing local growth
- Eliminate the risk of this deposit seeding distant sites.
- Provide an aesthetic result.

There has been a tendency to move away from radical operations to breast conservation. This has resulted from a realisation that prognosis is not altered greatly by more extensive excisions yet morbidity is increased.

Equally, for conservative surgery there has been a realisation that adjuvant radiotherapy to the breast is a necessity. Local recurrence rates of up to a third at 8 years occur in simple excision without radiotherapy. The rates with radiotherapy are between 10 and 20%.

Management of disease in the breast must be combined with a consideration of management of:

- Axillary disease
- Distant metastases.

Breast Conservation Surgery

Breast conservation surgery may involve either wide local excision or a quadrantectomy:

- Wide local excision involves removal of the tumour with at least a 1 cm margin of normal breast tissue.
- Quadrantectomy is more extensive and involves removal of a whole quadrant of the breast.

Breast conservation is often combined with axillary node dissection and/or local radiotherapy. The wider the excision the lower the recurrence rate, but the poorer the cosmetic result. However, cosmetic results are better generally than mastectomy and breast reconstruction is not usually required.

Alternative terms for operations involving breast conservation include lumpectomy, tumourectomy and tylectomy. They all imply removal of the tumour with a peripheral rim of normal tissue.

Breast tumours suitable for breast conservation include:

- Tumours where there is a single clinical and mammographic lesion.
- Tumour size:
  - less than 3-4 cm in diameter
  - dependent on the size of the breast:
    - § in small breasts, tumours greater than 2cm diameter may be impossible to remove without a cosmetic result that is similar to that of mastectomy.
    - § in large breasts, tumours slightly greater than 4cm diameter may be treated conservatively as the cosmetic results are generally favourable and prognosis is not thought to be greatly different from mastectomy.
- No sign of local advancement e.g. fixation to overlying skin or deeper muscle.

Mastectomy

A third of localised breast tumours are unsuitable for treatment by breast conservation. A number of procedures may be performed:

- Simple mastectomy:
  - removal of breast, nipple, areola and skin. Nodes may be removed separately. Chest wall muscles left intact
  - enables later reconstruction
- Modified radical mastectomy (Patey's operation):
  - removal of breast, nipple, areola, skin and level I and II axillary nodes plus pectoralis minor; pectoralis major muscle is preserved

Mutilating operations now rarely performed:

- Halsted radical mastectomy—removal of breast, nipple, areola, major and minor pectoralis muscles, axillary nodes

- Urban extended radical mastectomy—as above plus removal of internal mammary nodes, medial costal cartilages and part of sternum

The last two procedures are used only in advanced disease where their associated morbidity is less than that from radiotherapy

The tumours best treated with mastectomy include:

- Patient preference:
  - small tumours may be amenable to conservative treatment, but the patient may have a strong feeling that mastectomy will provide more peace of mind
  - patient may prefer to avoid radiotherapy with its attendant complications
- Size of tumour:
  - tumours greater than 2-3cm in small breasts; generally, removal of masses greater than this size results in a cosmetic defect that is unacceptable
  - in larger breasts, masses up to 4cm have been treated with breast conservation with little aesthetic deficit and what is believed to be little influence on prognosis
- Those with clinical or radiographic evidence of more than one tumour:
  - more prevalent with lobular carcinoma
  - multifocal disease:
    - § presence of synchronous tumour within the the same quadrant
    - § increases with increasing primary tumour size
    - § widespread multifocal disease is probably best treated with mastectomy.
  - multicentric disease: presence of synchronous tumour outside of the same quadrant
- Poor tumour differentiation

þ centrally-located tumours:

  - often difficult to excise by conservative measures without poor cosmesis due to loss of nipple

– many women prefer mastectomy to simple conservation if the nipple will be lost by both techniques.

Radiotherapy Treatment in Breast Cancer

Radiotherapy is commonly used in the management of breast cancer.

A meta-analysis has been shown that radiotherapy reduces the local recurrence rate by about two-thirds and significantly reduces breast cancer-related deaths (1).

However this study reveals that radiotherapy does increase other causes of death especially vascular disease—probably because the heart, coronaries and carotids are included in the irradiated field. Of note is that historical methods of radiation included overlapping fields, high daily doses, and larger irradiated volumes, all of which may increase mortality from causes other than breast cancer. This meta-analysis suggests that mortality from such causes may be lower when daily doses of < 2.2 Gy were employed.

This evidence suggests that many patients, especially those who are younger and node positive, should consider nodal irradiation, even when systemic treatment is given.

Systemic Treatments

Two types of systemic treatment are available:

- Hormonal therapy
- Cytotoxic chemotherapy

Hormonal therapy is best suited in the presence of slow growing disease, where the tumour is known to be oestrogen sensitive and since it is well tolerated it is ideal for elderly and unfit patients.

Cytotoxic chemotherapy is better suited where the tumour is rapidly progressive and when the tumour is oestrogen receptor negative.

Hormonal Therapy

Many breast cancer cells, particularly those which are oestrogen receptor positive require oestrogens to proliferate. Hormonal therapy aims to remove the proliferative oestrogen stimulus.

Hormonal therapy is used in two main circumstances:

- In advanced disease where surgery is not attempted or is not potentially curative
- In patients who have potentially curative surgery but who are at high risk of recurrence

Currently there are two approaches to reducing the oestrogen stimulus:

- Antioestrogens
- Aromatase inhibitors

Antioestrogens are used in the hormonal treatment of breast cancer. The gold standard is tamoxifen which is primarily an oestrogen receptor antagonist with some agonist acitivity.

Tamoxifen taken for 5 years following surgical treatment is a standard part of the treatment regime for postmenopausal women with hormone-receptor-positive breast cancer. If used in this context then tamoxifen:

- Increases the proportion of women who survive for at least 10 years from about 50% to 60% among those with lymph-node involvement
- Increases the proportion of women who survive for at least 10 years without lymph-node involvement from about 73% to 79%.
- Almost halves the risk of development of cancer in the contralateral breast.

Inhibition of aromatase prevents the synthesis of oestrogens.

Aminoglutethimide has been used in the past to produce a medical adrenalectomy, preventing the synthesis of adrenal oestrogens in patients post-oophorectomy. The clinically relevant activity of aminoglutethimide was aromatase inhibition. Recently specific inhibitors of aromatase have been developed which obviate the need for glucocorticoid replacement.

There are two classes of aromatase inhibitors:

- Non-steroidal:
  - anastozole
  - letrozole
  - are potent aromatase inhibitors which may be used in advanced breast cancer.
- Steroidal:
  - formestane
  - exemestane
  - may be used in advanced breast cancer.

Chemotherapy

Chemotherapy is indicated in two situations for the treatment of breast cancer:

- Adjuvant chemotherapy in patients at risk of micrometastasis.
- Treatment of known metastatic disease

First line treatment is with an anthracycline or mitozantrone. Resistant tumours may respond to a taxol compound.

Guidance from the National Institute of Clinical Excellence (NICE) states that both docetaxel (Taxotere) and paclitaxel (Taxol) should be available for the treatment of advanced breast cancer where initial cytotoxic chemotherapy (including anthracycline) has failed oris inappropriate.

Long Term follow-up

The aim of follow up is three fold:

- To detect local recurrence
- To detect disease in the other breast
- To ensure that a close eye is kept on first degree relatives particularly if the patient is pre-menopausal.

Regular clinical examination and mammography are recommended. Follow up should be arranged according to the type of surgery performed.

After breast conservation surgery, recurrence occurs at a fixed rate each year and the patient should be reviewed every 6 months. For mastectomy however, recurrence decreases with time and thus after 2 years of 6 monthly follow up, the patient may be reviewed annually.

Prognosis

Overall 5 year survival is 80%.
Influencing factors include:

- Clinical staging (manchester system):
  - stage 1—80% 5 year survival
  - stage 2—68% "
  - stage 3—40% "
  - stage 4—10% "
- Size—small i.e. less than 2 cm—95% 5 year survival;—large i.e. more than 2 cm—80% 5 year survival.
- Tumour type—tubular and mucinous have best prognosis.
- Grade—high grade tumours carry poorer prognosis.
- Receptor status—oestrogen receptor positive tumours are are more likely to respond to hormone therapy.
- Age at diagnosis.

Breast Cancer in the Male

Male breast cancer accounts 1% of all breast cancer. Among men with Klinefelter's syndrome, the incidence is comparable to that of women.

Presentation is usually in the 6th decade with a lump beneath the areola.

Management is similar to that in female breast carcinoma. Early disease is treated by surgery and radiotherapy; late disease, by hormonal therapy. Orchidectomy is often effective.

Breast cancer in men generally has a poorer prognosis than that in women. The smaller amount of breast tissue allows for a more rapid dissemination of metastases into regional lymphatics.

PAGET'S DISEASE OF THE NIPPLE

Paget's disease of the nipple is a presentation of breast cancer that invariably, is associated with ductal carcinoma in situ (DCIS) or invasive carcinoma in the underlying breast. Typically, it presents as a unilateral red, bleeding, eczematous lesion of the nipple which is eventually eroded.

This condition occurs in approximately 1 in 50 breast cancers, and is most frequent among middle-aged and elderly women.

About 40% of cases present with a palpable lump, a relatively late stage.

Rarely Paget's disease may affect other apocrine gland-bearing areas such as the vulva.

Histologic examination of the nipple reveals multiple Paget cells:

- Clear
- Sited among the basal epidermal cells
- Typical ballooned appearance
- Pale cytoplasm
- Prominent nuclei
- Nucleus surrounded by halo—accumulation of intracellular mucopolysaccharide.

At the skin, the epidermis is invaded. The underlying dermis contains an inflammatory infiltrate.

In the vast majority of cases, careful study of the breast reveals an associated DCIS or invasive carcinoma.

A popular theory is that Paget's disease results from invasion of the nipple by malignant cells spreading down the ducts from the associated breast tumour.

Other theories propose that the Paget cells arise in the nipple from local epidermal cells, and that the concurrence of DCIS and nipple malignant cells are due to common carcinogenic influences.

Clinical Features

Classically, the condition is unilateral. The earliest symptoms are those of itching, tingling and discomfort.

Later, a small patch of redness or roughening is evident on the nipple that progresses to frank erosion with red granulation tissue and bleeding. The areola is often affected. There may be a palpable lump.

Changes occur slowly. It may take 4-5 years for the nipple to be fully eroded.

Less commonly, Paget's disease is characterised by a dry, red, scaly rash that spreads widely to involve much of the breast.

Management is concentrated on detecting and treating any associated malignancy.

Total mastectomy with axillary dissection may be preferable in older patients as it is rapid and reliable. In those who wish to avoid mastectomy, radiotherapy alone or after cone excision of the nipple, areola and underlying ducts may be offered.

Wide local excision without radiotherapy is unsatisfactory; it is associated with a 50% recurrence rate. Adjuvant therapy is indicated only for established invasive carcinoma.

Paget's disease with associated intraduct carcinoma only and no palpable lump, has an excellent prognosis, with a cure rate approaching 100%.

Chapter 7

Pancreatic Diseases and Conditions

PANCREATITIS

Pancreatitis is an inflammatory disorder of the pancreas.

Acute pancreatitis varies in severity and may be life-threatening. Patients present with characteristic, acute abdominal pain.

Some experience persistent abdominal pain similar in nature to that of acute pancreatitis but without other the other associated features. The burden on the patient of this chronic pancreatitis should not be underestimated. It often persists for years before finally burning out.

A subgroup of patients suffer an initial acute attack followed by a prolonged relapsing and remitting clinical course. This type of chronic pancreatitis is known as chronic relapsing pancreatitis.

Chronic and acute pancreatitis are distinguished pathologically because 'in acute pancreatitis, the gland is normal before the attack and can return to normal after resolution of the attack, whereas in chronic pancreatitis , the gland is abnormal before or after the attack, or both.'

Acute Pancreatitis

Acute pancreatitis is the condition in which activated pancreatic enzymes leak into the substance of the pancreas and initiate the autodigestion of the gland.

It is relatively common and has shown a 10 fold increase in many Western countries in the last two decades. In the UK, about 250 per million population per year are affected. Alcohol is the most common cause in men; gallstones in women. AIDS patients are affected more commonly than other groups.

Acute pancreatitis accounts for approximately 1% of acute surgical admissions. Less than 10% of cases are severe enough to be life-threatening.

The condition is rare in children.

Aetiology

The most common causes of acute pancreatitis in adults are:

- Gallstones in the lower end of the common bile duct—45%
- Alcohol—35%
- Idiopathic—10%
- Miscellaneous e.g. hypertriglyceridaemia- 10%.

Pathogenesis

Acute pancreatitis is characterised by:

- Knflammation
- Proteolysis—from release of proteases
- Fat necrosis—from release of lipase and phospholipase.
- Haemorrhage—from release of elastase.

The activation of trypsin is thought to play a key role by:

- Activating other pro-enzymes in the acinar cells
- Activating the kinin system and initiating the clotting and complement systems

Three mechanisms are postulated:

- Acinar cell injury—causing release of intracellular pro-enzymes which are then activated. This may be the mechanism in acute pancreatitis associated with alcohol binging, viruses, drugs, ischaemia and trauma.

- Duct obstruction—a gallstone may impact at the ampulla and obstruct the pancreatic duct causing increased intraductal pressure and hence intercellular leakage of enzymes from small ducts into the interstitium. Alternatively, damage to the sphincter of Oddi allows reflux of duodenal contents into the pancreas. Lecithin in the refluxed material is converted by phospholipase A to lysolecithin which is highly toxic to acinar cells. In chronic alcoholism, acute attacks of pancreatitis may result from the precipitation of proteinaceous plugs in the pancreatic ducts which cause fibrosis and atrophy of the pancreas.
- Derangement in the intracellular transport of pancreatic enzymes—enzymes activated within the lysosomes by hydrolases.

Toxaemia results from the systemic absorption of enzymes and toxins. The sequestration of calcium into the areas of fat necrosis produces hypocalcaemia while the escape of large volumes of fluid into the peritoneal cavity results in hypovolaemic shock.

Clinical Features

Acute pancreatitis typically presents as an acute abdomen with the sudden onset of severe upper abdominal pain, often radiating to the back, nausea and vomiting. Once a chemical peritonitis is established, pain is felt throughout the abdomen and may be referred to the shoulder tip with involvement of the diaphragmatic peritoneum.

Early in the attack the patient may move around trying to find a comfortable position, obtaining relief by sitting forwards—the so-called "pancreatic position." Once generalised peritonitis supervenes, however, the patient remains still.

Other features are dependent upon the severity of the attack and the development of complications. Abdominal wall discolouration is almost pathognomonic and carries a mortality risk of about 40%.

Mild Acute Pancreatitis

The patient with mild pancreatitis looks well with no systemic features and minimal abdominal tenderness.

However, the pain may be considerable. It can be felt in a variety of places in the abdomen, most commonly centrally and in the epigastrium or right hypochondrium, but also in the left hypochondrium, and through to the back.

Moderate Acute Pancreatitis

The patient with moderate acute pancreatitis has a distended and diffusely tender abdomen with some guarding. After 12 to 24 hours, bowel sounds are absent due to an inflammatory ileus but hypovolaemia is less than in a severe attack and tachycardia may be the only systemic sign.

There may be mild jaundice due to periampullary oedema.

Severe Acute Pancreatitis

The patient with severe acute pancreatitis is still, grey and shocked.

Abdominal examination reveals signs of generalised peritonitis with extreme tenderness, guarding and rigidity. There is abdominal distension due to paralytic ileus and subcutaneous staining—in the flank (Grey-Turner's sign), peri-umbilical region (Cullen's sign), or less commonly, the infra-inguinal region (Fox's sign). Bowel sounds are absent.

Muscle twitches, cramps and spasm indicate hypocalcaemia.

The patient is hypovolaemic with sweating, tachycardia, and a decreased blood pressure and urinary output.

Investigations and Diagnosis

Blood tests:

- Serum amylase

- Serum lipase—usually elevated for longer than amylase.
- FBC—may reveal a leucocytosis and/or a rise in haemoglobin concentration due to haemoconcentration.
- Serum calcium—may be low due to sequestration of calcium in areas of fat necrosis.
- Urea and electrolytes—may show signs of dehydration.
- Liver function tests may be deranged with raised LDH, bilirubin and transaminases and low albumin.
- Blood glucose—may be high due to islet cell damage and destruction.
- CRP—helps discriminate mild and severe pancreatitis.
- Arterial gases—may show hypoxia and metabolic acidosis.

Imaging:

- Chest x-ray—may show elevation of the left hemidiaphragm with atelectasis and pleural effusion.
- Plain abdominal x-ray—may show a ground glass appearance due to the presence of a peritoneal exudate. Bowel gas is generally absent apart from a central dilated section of duodenum or jejunum known as a "sentinel" loop; it indicates localised ileus.
- Ultrasound—may detect a swollen gland, the presence of gallstones in the gallbladder, or dilatation of the common bile duct.
- CT—indicated if pancreas cannot be visualised by ultrasound. Often normal in mild attacks. If severe inflammation, pancreas is swollen and there is surrounding oedema.

Stool examination—may reveal unsuspected gallstones.

Peritoneal lavage—confirms the diagnosis if an odourless, yellow-brown, amylase-rich fluid is aspirated. May relieve pain and avoid unnecessary laparotomy.

Treatment

Initial treatment is essentially supportive. During the first 24 hours, blood pressure, urine volume, pulse and respiratory rate, are checked hourly, and temperature and blood glucose, 4-6 hourly. Oral intake is withheld to rest the pancreas and the bowel. Nasogastric suction is given to reduce vomiting and abdominal distension.

Analgesia is essential. Opiates are preferred, usually, pethidine, i.m.; morphine is avoided as it constricts the sphincter of Oddi. NSAID's are avoided because of the increased risk of GI bleeding and renal dysfunction.

Ranson Criteria in Acute Pancreatitis

The initial clinical picture is not a reliable indicator of future events in mild pancreatitis. Patients with seemingly mild disease may deteriorate rapidly and die.

The Ranson criteria and other severity scoring systems, e.g. Glasgow, APACHE II, enable early diagnosis of severe acute pancreatitis. This can be defined as the presence of three or more of the following criteria within 48 hours of admission:

- Age above than 55 years
- Blood glucose above 10 mmol/L—no history of diabetes
- White cell count above 15 x 10^9 / L
- LDH above 600 IU/L
- Aspartate transaminase above 200 u/L
- Corrected calcium less than 2.0 mmol/L
- Blood urea above 16 mmol/L—no improvement with intravenous fluids
- Decreasing haematocrit
- Arterial pO2 less than 8 kPa (60 mm Hg)
- Metabolic acidosis
- Serum albumin less than 32 g/L.

N.B. the serum amylase value is not one of the criteria.

The mortality per postive criterion:

- NUMBER OF POSITIVE CRITERIA
  - 0-2 <5% mortality
  - 3-4 20% mortality
  - 5-6 40% mortality
  - 7-8 100% mortality.

Complications

Intra-abdominal:

- Pancreatic "collections":
  - phlegmon
  - pseudocyst
  - abscess
  - necrosis.
- Intestinal:
  - paralytic ileus
  - gastrointestinal haemorrhage—from stress ulceration, gastric varices due to splenic vein obstruction, or rupture of pseudoaneurysm
  - necrotising obstruction or fistulisation of colon.
- Hepatic—obstructive jaundice due to oedematous narrowing of common bile duct.
- Renal—hydronephrosis and hydroureter of right kidney due to peripancreatic inflammation in peri-renal space.
- Spleen—rupture or haematoma, from spread of peripancreatic inflammation.

Systemic complications range from minor pyrexia to rapidly fatal, multiple organ-system failure. They include:

- Circulatory shock—kinin activation, haemorrhage.
- Disseminated intravascular coagulation.
- Respiratory insufficiency:
  - Mild e.g. hypoxaemia, atelectasis, pleural effusion
  - Severe e.g. adult respiratory distress syndrome.
- Acute renal failure

- Metabolic:
  - hypocalcaemia
  - hyperglycaemia/diabetes mellitus
  - hypertriglyceridaemia
- Pancreatic encephalopathy—confusions, delusions, coma.
- Retinal arteriolar obstruction causing sudden blindness.
  - Purtscher's retinopathy
- Metastatic fat necrosis.

Prognosis

Mortality from acute pancreatitis ranges from 1% in mild attacks to 50% in severe attacks to almost 100% in patients with multiple complications and poor prognostic signs.

To prevent recurrence, the cause should be identified and eradicated. Cholecystectomy should be performed during the same admission if gallstones are suspected, as this is safer than delaying for 3 months. Alcohol should be screened by taking a careful history from the patient and relatives or close friends. Neither plasma gamma glutamyl transpeptidase nor blood alcohol are reliable indicators of abuse. Sadly, advice to abstain is rarely heeded.

Most investigators do not believe that chronic pancreatitis results for acute pancreatitis unless complications such as pseudocysts or ductal strictures are present.

Pancreatic Pseudocyst

A pancreatic pseudocyst is a localised collection of pancreatic juice. It may be within, adjacent to, or remote from the pancreas—ie intrasplenic or mediastinal.

Pancreatic pseudocysts are formed by pancreatic secretions escaping from a ruptured duct, and do not have an epithelial lining. Occasionally they contain small amounts of necrotic debris. Persistence of the pseudocyst indicates continuing communication with the duct.

Typically, acute pancreatitis causes pseudocyst formation in 50% of cases with first symptoms evolving four weeks after the episode.

The pseudocyst may:

- Resolve
- Enlarge, causing pain and biliary or pyloric obstruction.
- Become infected, forming an abscess.
- Rupture into the peritoneum, leading to ascites.
- Erode a vessel, causing severe haemorrhage.

Clinical Features

Pancreatic pseudocysts have the following points of interest in the history:

- Severe epigastric pain
- Epigastric fullness
- Nausea and vomiting
- Systemic manifestations of cyst infection—sweating, fever, rigors
- recent history of acute pancreatitis.

On examination

- With large cysts, a mass is felt above the umbilicus that is fixed, tender and classically, tense. Its borders may be hard to define.
- Smaller cysts are commonly impalpable.

Management

A high index of suspicion must be maintained for the occurrence of a pseudocyst in subjects with a recent history of acute pancreatitis. Confirmation and follow-up is obtained with CT, or more practically, with ultrasound scanning.

Up to 40% of acute pseudocysts will resolve within approximately one week. Supportive treatment is all that is required in this time.

Should the cyst fail to resolve after 2 months, become infected, or is greater than 6cm in diameter, cystogastrostomy or cystojejunostomy is required. The former entails:

- Entering the anterior wall of the stomach.
- Fashioning a large hole through the posterior wall into the pseudocyst.
- Securing stomach and pseudocyst with a circumferential stitch.

The pseudocyst then drains into the stomach.

Pancreatic Abscess

A pancreatic abscess is a well-encapsulated collection of liquid pus, in or around the pancreas. It denotes an end stage of pancreatic inflammation when infection supervenes. Necrotic debris initially results from the action of pancreatic enzymes and then becomes the focus of bacterial infection.

Patients usually present with a swinging pyrexia and tachycardia, several weeks after an attack of acute pancreatitis. The diagnosis is confirmed with ultrasound and CT, and with aspiration of pus.

Surgical drainage and removal of necrotic debris is indicated. A drain is placed under CT guidance. Percutaneous drainage is hindered by viscosity, loculation and retroperitoneal tracking. In severe cases, conventional surgical operation is required.

Chronic Pancreatitis

Chronic pancreatitis is characterised by irreversible glandular destruction and permanent loss of endocrine and exocrine function. It may follow episodes of acute pancreatitis or may occur without an identifiable attack.

The incidence is increasing. In the UK, about 5 new cases are reported annually per 100,000 of the population. The most common aetiological agent is alcohol but in some patients, no satisfactory explanation is available.

Aetiology

Alcohol accounts for up to 80% of all cases of chronic pancreatitis. Other causes include:

- Congenital—pancreas divisum; annular pancreas
- Hereditary—sometimes with cyclical neutropenia
- Cystic fibrosis—in young adults
- Hypercalcaemia
- Hyperlipidaemia
- Obstruction of the pancreatic duct can cause chronic pancreatitis.
  - mechanical or structural changes of the pancreatic—duct sphincter, pseudocysts, post—traumatic ductal strictures, periampullary tumours.
  - gallstones is an uncommon cause.
  - a pancreas divisum is a very rare cause.
- Idiopathic—30—40% of patients; tend to cluster in two groups—a younger group (with peak incidence of 15—30 years of age) and an older group (peak of 50—70 years).

Morphology

Morphological patterns commonly seen in chronic pancreatitis include:

- Chronic calcifying pancreatitis—an irregular, lobular, spotty distribution of calcification within the pancreatic parenchyma. The acini are atrophic with increased interlobular fibrous tissue. Pseudocyst formation is common. This pattern is usually seen in alcoholics.
- Chronic obstructive pancreatitis—with inflammation of varying severity to the left of the obstruction and normal or near normal pancreas to the right. Calcification is rare and protein plugs are uncommon. The changes are more prominent in the head of the pancreas. This pattern is usually seen in cases associated with congenital anomalies or previous acute inflammation.

- Minimal change—changes are microscopic, in the acinar architecture, rather than macroscopically. Usually follows an attack of proven acute pancreatitis.
- Phlegmon
- Pseudocyst
- Abscess.

Clinical Features

Severe disease may develop before symptoms are evident. In the West most patients have a history of prolonged and heavy alcohol use.

Clinical features of chronic pancreatitis may include:

- Abdominal pain—mainly epigastric and upper abdominal; may radiate to the back. The pain is variable and may be severe. It may be continuous and difficult to distinguish from that of pancreatic carcinoma; or may be episodic, often, but not always, precipitated by alcohol.
- Anorexia and weight loss—due to malabsorption and/or small meals.
- Features of exocrine insufficiency:
  - steatorrhoea—occurs in about 50% of patients; can be minimal in patients who reduce their fat intake
  - hypocalcaemia—unabsorbed fat chelates calcium
  - malabsorption of fat—but malabsorption of fat soluble vitamins rarely produces symptoms such as bleeding tendency
  - protein catabolism—protein malabsorption due to deficiency of pancreatic proteases—exacerbates weight loss.
- Features of endocrine insufficiency:
  - impaired glucose tolerance
  - eventually, frank diabetes.
- Other features:
  - obstructive jaundice.

- portal hypertension from splenic or portal vein thrombosis
- pancreatic duct strictures.

Examination reveals epigastric tenderness; rarely, a mass.

Investigation

The salient investigations in chronic pancreatitis include:

- Blood tests:
  - serum amylase—usually normal but may be mildly raised in an acute on chronic attack
  - albumin and clotting studies—may be abnormal due to associated cirrhosis or malabsorption
  - low calcium or serum vitamin B_{12} suggests malabsorption
  - elevated alkaline phosphatase suggests biliary tract obstruction if gamma GT is raised, or rarely, osteomalacia
  - glucose may be raised if exocrine insufficiency.
- Imaging:
  - abdominal x-ray—30% show pancreatic calcification in later stages.
  - ultrasound—reveals gallstones, duct dilatation, pancreatic morphology.
  - CT scan—indicated if ultrasound is abnormal; shows major abnormalities in pancreatic anatomy.
  - ERCP—"gold standard"; reveals duct dilatation and distortion of main pancreatic duct and side branches; however, a normal ERCP does not absolutely exclude chronic pancreatitis.
- Functional tests—e.g. secretin, Lundh, pancreolauryl tests—useful in the diagnosis of patients who have recurrent symptoms and whose imaging and other tests are normal.

Differential Diagnosis

Chronic pancreatitis must be differentiated from pancreatic carcinoma, usually on the basis of ultrasound or CT. Other potentially useful tests for differentiation of these conditions include cytologic examination of pancreatic—duct fluid, fine needle biopsy of the pancreas, and measurement of tumour markers for pancreatic carcinoma e.g. carcinoembryonic antigen and CA19-9 (although these are not pathognomic for pancreatic cancer).

Treatment Modalities

The underlying cause should be identified and treated. Complete abstinence from alcohol is required. In the absence of life-threatening complications or malignancy, conservative management is preferred. Severely ill patients may require a period of in-patient management. Those who are less ill may be managed as out-patients. Blood levels for alcohol should be taken in those who relapse.

Medical

Exocrine insufficiency may be treated by a combination of a low-fat diet and pancreatic enzyme supplements, e.g. creon, pancrease.

Endocrine insufficiency may be treated by diet, oral hypoglycaemics or insulin as appropriate. Control may be difficult to achieve as patients may experience severe hypoglycaemia due to a lack of glucagon.

Pain relief may be achieved by abstinence from alcohol or enzyme supplementation. Specific measures include codeine; pethidine—but risk of dependence if used long term; and referral to pain clinic. *Morphine is not recommended* as it constricts the sphincter of Oddi. However, in severe paroxysms, its potent analgesia may outweigh any risks of obstruction.

Surgical

Surgery may be considered if ERCP demonstrates localised chronic pancreatitis or focal lesions, e.g.

calculi; it may also be considered for intractable pain, pancreatic cysts and pseudocysts, and recurrent gastrointestinal haemorrhage.

Options include:

- Cholecystectomy with clearance of duct stones—essential if gallstones present
- Sphincterotomy of the accessory papilla in patients with pancreas divisum
- Drainage—longitudinal pancreatojejunostomy in patients whose pancreatic duct is 8 mm or more in diameter; percutaneous or surgical drainage of a pseudocyst or abscess
- Partial resection—body and tail may be resected if pathology is limited to them. In other patients, a **Whipple's procedure** may be necessary.
- Total pancreatectomy—if all other therapy has failed.

Prognosis

The prognosis of chronic pancreatitis is dependent on age and adherence to medical therapy such as abstinence from alcohol.

Chronic pancreatitis may burn out after many years as the gland atrophies and malabsorption and diabetes develop. Overall, about 25-30% die within 10 years. Pancreatic cancer develops in approximately 4% of patients with a 20 year history of chronic pancreatitis

Pancreatic Carcinoma

A disease of later life, pancreatic carcinoma is the third most common cancer of the gastrointestinal tract and the sixth most common cause of cancer deaths.

Seventy percent of tumours occur in the head of the pancreas in proportion to the amount of tissue in different parts of the pancreas.

Progress is insidious. There is early regional lymph node involvement and spread to the liver. The tumour may metastasize to bone and lung.

Less common endocrine tumours of the pancreas such as glucagonomas and insulinomas may occur.

Aetiology

The cause of pancreatic carcinoma is unknown.

Factors which have been associated with the development of pancreatic carcinoma include:

- Smoking
- Chronic pancreatitis, possibly secondary to alcohol consumption
- High fat diet, which may explain the rising incidence in affluent countries
- Diabetes mellitus

Certain industries seem to impart a high risk to their workers; occupational exposure to coal gas and aluminium increase the risk.

Coffee consumption is no longer considered to be a risk factor.

Clinical Features

Presenting features of pancreatic carcinoma include:

- Weight loss in 80%.
- Deep epigastric pain, which in 60% of cases, radiates to the back. It is a very hard pain to treat.
- Jaundice with pruritis if tumour affects head of the pancreas and obstructs the biliary system; occurs in 50%.
- Ascites with a knobbly liver in 30%.
- Anorexia, nausea, vomiting.
- Palpable gallbladder—Courvoisier's law.

Less common presentations:

- Steatorrhoea.
- Thrombophlebitis migrans: may also occur in glucagonomas.
- Acute pancreatitis.
- Gastric outlet obstruction, causing pyloric stenosis.
- Gastrointestinal haemorrhage due to duodenal erosion.

- Symptoms of hypoglycaemia may occur if the tumour is an insulinoma—very rare.

Investigations

- Biochemistry:
  - raised serum bilirubin and alkaline phosphatase in obstructive jaundice
  - may be impaired glucose tolerance or diabetes.
- Ultrasound—to look for dilated ducts and stones .
- ERCP or transhepatic percutaneous cholangiography.
  - allows a pancreatogram to be taken
  - pancreatic juice can be collected for cytology.
- CT scan—the most reliable method of diagnosis—may show metastatic disease.
- CT or US guided biopsy—may be used to confirm the diagnosis.
- carcinoembryonic antigen—may be raised if hepatic metastases.

Management of Pancreatic Carcinoma

The management of pancreatic carcinoma can be divided into steps able to cure or palliate:

- *Curative:* surgery offers the only possibility of cure. A radical pancreaticoduodenectomy—Whipple's operation—may be used in this condition. Surgery should be performed in specialist centres. There is evidence that surgery plus adjuvant therapy with 5-fluoruracil, alone or in combination, may prolong survival (from around 11-14 months to 20-23 months) but this requires confirmation (1).
- Palliative:
  - jaundice and associated itching can be relieved by procedures such as endoscopic or percutaneous stenting. Surgical intervention requires the creation of a biliary diversion via a cholecystojejunostomy.
  - vomiting may be due to duodenal involvement and thus a gastroenterostomy may be necessary

– pain relief is achieved using opiates and/or coeliac plexus block.
– chemotherapy (1)—for patients with advanced disease, gemcitabine is easily administered in the outpatient setting, is relatively well tolerated, and is a useful first-line treatment in patients able to manage most, or all, self-care. However, the overall treatment benefits are limited.

Prognosis

The prognosis of pancreatic carcinoma is very poor. Without surgical treatment, less than 3% of all patients survive for 5 years.

The benefit of surgical intervention is dependent on the site of the tumour. A Whipple's resection for carcinoma of the head of the pancreas can give, at best, a 5-year survival of 19%. An absence of lymph node involvement was associated with an improved prognosis. Tumours of the body and tail of the pancreas are associated with a worse prognosis, whatever the mode of intervention, 1-year survival was 8-9%.

Glucagonoma

This is a result of a tumour of the alpha 2 cells of the islets of Langerhans. The majority of these tumours are malignant.

This tumour may present with attacks of hyperglycaemia, stomatitis, vulvitis, anaemia, a rash and diarrhoea. Necrolytic migratory erythema is specifically associated with this condition.

This tumour forms of part of a multiple endocrine neoplasia syndrome (MEN I).

Insulinoma

This is a result of a tumour of the APUD cells of the islets of Langerhans. The majority of these APUD tumours are benign.

The most common of these rare tumours is an insulinoma which are derived from beta cells. This tumour may present with attacks of hypoglycaemia, especially when fasting and exercising. Attacks are treated with oral or intravenous glucose. The vast majority (90%) are benign.

Diagnosis is based on:

- Inappropriate hyperinsulinaemia
- High ratio of proinsulin to insulin in a fasting blood sample (due to defective post-translational processing of proinsulin which allows proinsulin to be secreted in addition to insulin and C-peptide).
- CT scanning and/or pancreatic arteriography to identify the site of the lesion—usually in distal 2/3 of pancreas (occasionally in head of pancreas or ectopic site such as duodenal wall).

This tumour forms of part of a multiple endocrine neoplasia syndrome (MEN I).

Management: surgery or medical treatment with diazoxide.

Chapter

8

Gastrointestinal Diseases and Conditions

MOUTH AND THROAT DISEASE

Cancrum Oris

Cancrum oris is a quickly advancing gangrene of the lips and cheeks. It is associated with a mixed bacterial infection which includes Borrelia vincentii.

It may be seen in:

- Measles:
  - especially in the malnourished, typically in children in tropical Africa
  - cranium oris develops from an acute, ulcerative gingivitis
- Leukaemic patients:
  - often a terminal complicaton of the disease
  - associated with the use of anti-inflammatory and immunosuppressive drugs

Ranula

A Ranula is a transparent retention cyst in the floor of the mouth arising from the sublingual salivary glands. Ranula means a small frog and the cyst is so-called because of a supposed resemblance to a small frog.

The cyst enlarges slowly, penetrating the deep structures of the floor of the mouth above the mylo-hyoid muscle. It is more common in neonates and children and potentially can cause respiratory embarrassment. It appears as a blue-grey, dome-like swelling beneath the tongue. It may burst spontaneously, discharging its contents and collapsing, but almost invariably recurring.

Treatment depends on size. Small ranulae are excised; larger ones are marsupialized, i.e. de-roofed so that the cyst opens into the floor of the mouth.

Sublingual Dermoid Cyst

This is a developmental abnormality which may present as a swelling in the neck.

A sublingual dermoid cyst may be above or below the hyoid bone.

Sublingual Gland Tumour

Salivary gland tumours may be benign or malignant and are divided into:

- Tumours of the major salivary glands:
  - parotid
  - submandibular
  - sublingual
- Tumours of the minor salivary glands:
  - oral mucosa
  - palate
  - uvula
  - floor of mouth
  - posterior tongue
  - retromolar area
  - peritonsillar area
  - pharynx
  - larynx
  - paranasal sinuses

Benign Tumours of Salivary Glands

Pleomorphic adenomas are the most common benign tumours of salivary glands followed by Warthin's tumour. Rarer types include oncocytomas and monomorphic adenomas.

They usually present as a slowly growing lump. Most affect the parotid region. True malignant transformation may take place, especially in tumours of minor salivary tissue. If malignancy is suspected, the tissue should be biopsied so that appropriate, definitive treatment can be planned.

Pleomorphic Adenoma of the Salivary Gland

A pleomorphic adenoma is the most common neoplasm of the salivary glands, accounting for 50% of all salivary gland tumours, and for 70% of all parotid tumours.

Ninety percent occur in the parotid. The remainder are found in the submandibular, sublingual, or accessory salivary glands. Most present in middle age or later but any age may be affected. They are slightly more common in women than in men. It is the most common cause of a lump in the parotid or submandibular gland.

This tumour is regarded as benign but lacks true encapsulation, may infiltrate surrounding tissue, and may recur. The less differentiated tumours may be difficult to distinguish from frank carcinoma, and may metastasize to cervical lymph nodes or less commonly, through the blood stream to the lungs.

A pleomorphic adenoma usually presents as an asymptomatic, lump, which has been slowly enlarging for several years over or just behind the angle of the mandible. The vast majority occur in patients below the age of 50 years. Men and women are affected equally.

They are commonly found in the lower pole of the parotid gland.

Notably, pain and tenderness are absent. The lesion may be of any size and is usually firm. It is not fixed to overlying structures or mucosa.

Pleomorphic adenomas may become very large yet still do not affect the facial nerve. Any facial weakness implies malignancy.

Enucleation of a pleomorphic adenoma is inadequate. Treatment is by wide excision of the tumour and surrounding tissue with careful preservation of the facial nerve. This may be followed by radiotherapy, especially in elderly patients. The treatment must be applied to all salivary glands involved.

Following excision, prognosis is good but inadequate surgery often is followed by.

Warthin's Tumour

A Warthin's tumour is a benign tumour that occurs almost exclusively in the parotid glands, primarily in the tail. It accounts for about 5% of all parotid tumours. Ten percent occur bilaterally. It usually arises after middle age, with a male:female ratio of 5:1. There is a strong association with smoking.

It is composed of large glandular acini, embedded in dense lymphoid tissue in which lymphoid follicles may be seen. It is thought to arise from the salivary duct epithelium, the lymphoid tissue originating from the lymphoid aggregates present in the normal parotid gland.

The tumour presents as a soft, cystic lump. It alone, among salivary neoplasms, will concentrate technetium 99m. Warthin tumours are said to exude a highly-characteristic yellow or brown fluid if damaged.

Treatment is by superficial parotidectomy. Recurrence is rare but a satellite lesion may enlarge and present as another tumour. Prognosis after operation is good.

Recurrence.

Malignant Salivary Gland Tumours

Malignant salivary gland tumors are divided histologically into low-grade and high-grade malignancies:

- Low-grade malignancies:
  - acinic cell tumors
  - mucoepidermoid carcinoma (grades I or II)

- High-grade malignancies:
  - mucoepidermoid carcinoma (grade III)
  - adenocarcinoma:
    - § poorly differentiated carcinoma
    - § anaplastic carcinoma
  - squamous cell carcinoma
  - malignant mixed tumours
  - adenoid cystic carcinoma

The malignant tumours commonly affecting the major salivary glands include:

- Mucoepidermoid carcinoma.
- Acinic cell carcinoma.
- Adenoid cystic carcinoma, and less frequently.
- Primary squamous cell carcinomas.
- Pleomorphic adenomas, often derived from benign neoplasms.

Among minor salivary glands:

- Adenoid cystic carcinoma is the most common
- Adenocarcinoma.
- Mucoepidermoid carcinoma.

OESOPHAGEAL DISEASES AND CONDITIONS

Achalasia

Achalasia is a neuromuscular failure of relaxation at the lower end of the oesophagus with progressive dilatation, tortuosity, incoordination of peristalsis and often hypertrophy of the oesophagus above. There is effectively a functional obstruction at the lower end of the oesophagus.

Achalasia may occur at any age but particularly in the third to fourth decades. Males and females are affected equally.

Incidence is about 1 per 100,000 per year.

The **clinical features** of achalasia include:

- Gradually progressive, intermittent dysphagia; the dysphagia associated with oesophageal carcinoma is more rapid and relentless than achalasia. The insidious onset and progression prevents early presentation.

- Regurgitation of fluids from the oesophageal sac may be followed by an aspiration pneumonia or frank vomiting; the patient may have a history of recurrent respiratory tract infections
- Dysphagia is more marked for solids than liquids
- There may be an associated hiatus hernia
- The patient may advance to a state of debilitation due to chronic malnourishment.

Achalasia can occur at any age, but its greatest incidence is between 30 and 40 with both sexes being affected equally.

Investigations are as follows:

- Barium swallow—characteristic appearance with proximal dilatation and distal smooth tapering.
- manometric tests—demonstrate the motility disorder.
- oesophagoscopy—exclusion of carcinoma.

A chest radiograph may reveal:

- Widened mediastinum with possibly a fluid level behind the heart
- Absence of a gastric air bubble.

Manometric studies reveal a gastro-oesophageal sphincter that has a high resting tone and only partially relaxes. The tone does not fall to gastric fundal pressure.

The **differential diagnosis** of oesophageal achalasia includes:

- Oesphageal carcinoma
- Vigorous achalasia.

Management

Achalasia is incurable. However, treatment can be directed at relief of the distal obstruction.

- Pharmacological treatment—intrasphincteric injection of botulinum toxin should be considered as the initial therapy for patients with idiopathic achalasia who are at high risk for the complications of pneumatic dilatation or surgical myotomy.

- Endoscopic hydrostatic or pneumatic dilatation—this is with a balloon on the end of an endoscope, repeated monthly.
- Heller's operation—cardiomyotomy—cut distal 3 to 4 cm of oesophageal muscle longitudinally; the operation has a success rate of about 90% in those who do not respond to dilatation.

Both of the latter two treatments may produce subsequent reflux oesophagitis.

Dilatation has a lower mortality, but there is a potential complication of perforation in 2%. Overall, it is very successful, and it is used as a first line treatment with the 10% that fail going on to surgery.

The **complications** of oesophageal achalasia include:

- Aspiration pneumonia
- Haemorrhage
- Oesophageal carcinoma.

Barrett's oesophagus

Barrett's oesophagus is a condition in which there is gastric or intestinal metaplasia of the mucosa of the distal oesophagus.

Although it may rarely be congenital in origin, Barrett's oesophagus is most often an acquired condition and represents an important complication of long-standing gastro-oesophageal reflux. In acquired Barrett's oesophagus, chronic gastro-oesophageal reflux causes the squamous mucosa of the oesphagus to undergoe metaplastic change. This process appears to cause the squamocolumnar junction (ora serrata) to migrate caudally.

Barrett's oesophagus is most common in elderly adults, but is also seen in children and even in infants under two years of age.

Possible Clinical Features include:

- Dyspepsia
- Dysphagia
- Vomiting
- Haemetemesis
- Melaena
- Retrosternal pain that radiates to the neck (worsened after hot or cold foods).

Barrett's oesophagus is defined as columnar metaplasia of the oesophageal mucosa which ranges more than 2 cm from the gastro-oesophgeal junction. This condition may affect the whole of the oesophagus.

Endoscopic visualisation and biopsy are diagnostic.

The management of Barrett's oesophagus is controversial.

If pre-malignant changes are identified then some advocate oesophageal resection (particularly in fit, younger patients). Others advocate the use of regular endoscopy monitoring and intensive anti-reflux measures (long term proton pump inhibitor therapy and laser ablation of the site of metaplasia).

Barrett's oesophagus may be complicated by:

- Ulceration—Barrett's ulcer
- Stricture formation
- Adenocarcinoma of the oesophagus.

Boerhaave's Syndrome

Boerhaave's syndrome is the spontaneous rupture of a non-diseased oesophagus, usually after vigorous vomiting. It is associated with excessive alcohol ingestion when a dramatically raised pressure may develop in the oesophagus as a result of failure of cricopharyngeal relaxation. It is vital to recognise early because of its fatal consequences.

It is very rare and was first described by Herman Boerhaave in 1724.

The clinical symptoms of Boerhaave's syndrome include:

- Characteristically seen in middle aged men with a history of high alcohol intake, 'retching' and vomiting.
- Often give a history of retrosternal pain progressing to to excruciating epigastric pain that is increased by swallowing.
- Failure of opiates to relieve pain.

Signs of Boerhaave's syndrome include:

- Respiratory collapse:
  - dyspnoea
  - cyanosis
  - shock.
- Subcutaneous emphysema in the neck
- Hydrothorax } take some hours
- Pneumothorax } to develop
- Pleural effusion
- Tenderness over epigastrium and rigidity.

The differential diagnosis of Boerhaave's syndrome includes:

- Acute pancreatitis
- Acute cholecystitis
- Pulmonary embolism
- Myocardial infarction
- Dissecting aortic aneurysm
- Gastroduodenal perforation.

The diagnosis of Boerhaave's syndrome is made after:

- Chest X-ray:
  - after a few hours, air and fluid in the pleural cavity
  - mediastinal emphysema
- *Contrast studies:* definitive diagnosis made with gastrograffin swallow to show the site of the perforation
- CT scanning.

The treatment of Boerhaave's syndrome is surgical. Ideally, this should be instituted within six hours of diagnosis and with stabilization of the patient: after this time, the metabolic effects and damage to the oesophagus make survival less likely.

Surgery entails draining the pleural cavity, searching for concomitant pathology at thoracotomy, e.g. tumours, oversewing the lesion, and closing the chest with an underwater seal drain. Oesophagectomy may be required for extensive stenosing lesions. Parenteral feeding or a feeding gastrostomy may be required.

Surgery has a 36% mortality, whereas medical management has a 65% mortality within 24 hours and a 100% mortality after one week.

But note, Larrieu et al. report of one case which was treated sucessfully with medical therapy.

Oesophageal Carcinoma

Oesophageal carcinoma is becoming more common, unlike the trend observed in gastric carcinoma. It is most strongly linked to alcohol, especially spirits, and smoking.

Physical signs are rare apart from wasting and perhaps a palpable supraclavicular node. The principal symptom is dysphagia.

Patients are often able to locate the level of the obstruction in their oesophagus quite accurately. For example, a carcinoma of the oesophagus in its lower third will be a described as a feeling of a blockage behind the lower part of the sternum.

Tumours tend to arise in areas of partial narrowing, i.e. at the pharyngo-oesophageal junction (40%); the junction of the upper and middle third (40%); and where the oesophagus passes through the diaphragm (20%).

Aetiology

The principle aetiological factor appears to be chronic local tissue irritation.

Possible risk factors for oesophageal cancer include:

- Alcohol
- Smoking
- Achalasia
- Caustic stricture of the oesophagus
- Geographical location e.g. China and Northern Iran
- Barrett's oesophagus
- Plummer-Vinson syndrome
- Coeliac disease
- Tylosis—hyperkeratosis of the palms and soles.

Squamous carcinomas form the majority of cancers in the proximal and middle third of the oesophagus.

Adenocarcinomas are more likely to occur in the lower third of the oesophagus and are associated with chronic gastro-oesophageal reflux and the change to columnar epithelium associated with this.

Pathology

An oesophageal carcinoma commences as a nodule which then develops into either a papilliferous mass (60%), an ulcer (25%), or an annular constriction, usually of the cardia.

Historically, the large majority of oesophageal carcinomata were squamous. Today the incidence of adenocarcinoma is rising rapidly and now accounts for 50% of all oesophageal carcinomata in the USA.

Squamous carcinoma typically arises in the upper two thirds of the oesophagus. Adenocarcinoma usually arises in a region of specialised columnar epithelium (SCE) metaplasia in the lower third of the oesophagus—Barrett's oesophagus.

DISTRIBUTION FREQUENCY % CELL TYPE
Cervical 10 squamous upper third 20 squamous middle third 20 squamous lower third 50 90% adenocarcinoma

Staging

The staging of oesophageal carcinoma is important in order to try to prevent unnecessary surgical intervention.

There are several complimentary means of determining the stage:

- Chest radiography
- Barium swallow
- Ultrasound examination
- CT and MRI scanning
- Bronchoscopy

Given the data from these techniques, the tumour can be sited on the following standard scale:

- *Stage I:* limited to oesophagus and less than 5 cm in length
- *Stage II:* limited to oesophagus, greater than 5 cm in length and with resectable nodes
- *Stage III:* lesion greater than 10 cm in length, extension through oesophagus into adjacent structures, inoperable nodes or inoperable lesion.
- *Stage IV:* lesion as in stage III with evidence of perforation, fistula or distant metastasis.

Clinical Features

Dysphagia is the most frequently presented feature of oesophageal carcinoma:

- The patient may recount a short history of progressive dysphagia, initially affecting solids only, but gradually affecting the swallowing of fluids.
- The interruption of the passage of food may cause the individual to slowly alter the diet from solid to liquid nutrition; success with this approach may be at the expense of early medical self-referral.
- The level at which difficulty in swallowing is encountered may be identifiable by the patient.
- A short history of dysphagia in an elderly male is almost certainly carcinoma of the oesophagus or the cardia of the stomach.
- An infrequent presentation is of the obstruction of a large bolus of food with no prior history of dysphagia.

Other local features may include:

- Regurgitation of food or blood-stained vomit

- Aspiration pneumonia
- Pain:
  - classically, retrosternally and in the interscapular region
  - it may radiate to the jaws and arms.

General manifestations of malignant disease may include:

- Loss of weight, due to the metabolic effects of the tumour and a reduced intake of food
- Anorexia
- Anaemia
- Coughing, due to regurgitation or a fistula
- Oedema, due to a severe reduction in protein intake in the late stages.

Secondary deposits occur in:

- Lymph nodes
- In the liver causing jaundice.

Diagnosis

The diagnosis of oesophageal carcinoma is made on:

- History and examination
- Barium swallow:
  - the first-line investigation after the history of dysphagia
  - characteristic image of an irregular stricture with shouldered margins, 4-10 cm long and often tortuous
  - a tracheo-oesophageal fistula may also be demonstrated.
- Endoscopy and biopsy:
  - establishes histology and limits of lesion
  - can be used therapeutically to dilate, so improving nutrition before a definitive operative intervention.
- Cytology by washing/abrasion technique—used for screening in China.
- CT scanning helps to determine mediastinal involvement and whether metastasis has occurred to the liver.

- Bronchoscopy may be needed to exclude bronchial involvement in upper and middle-third lesions.
- Ultrasound may be used to identify secondary liver deposits.

Management

Management of oesophageal carcinoma is dependent on the level of the lesion and the stage of the disease.

Upper third lesion—high dose radiotherapy is indicated for lesions up to 5 cm long. Vital structures in the mediastinum closely related to the upper third make surgical clearance and resection very difficult.

Middle third lesion—early tumours are resectable. Again, radical radiotherapy may be indicated if the lesion is up to 5 cm long.

Lower third lesion—most accessible surgically; adenocarcinomas are radioresistant.

Extensive disease requires palliation of dysphagia:

- Endoscopic laser surgery for lesions less than 8 cm long.
- Oesophageal stenting—e.g. with a Celestin tube—if longer than 8 cm.
- Alternatives include:
  - oesophago-gastrostomy or oesophago-jejunostomy
  - short course radiotherapy.

Prognosis

The prognosis for oesophageal carcinoma is dependent on the site of the tumour. Approximate 5-year survival figures are:

- Upper third tumours have a 20% 5-year survival.
- Middle third tumours have a 6% 5-year survival.
- Lower third tumours have a 15% 5-year survival.

The prognosis also depends on:

- Tumour size and site
- Depth of invasion
- Node metastases

- Widespread metastases
- Tumour grade
- Lymphocytic response
- General health of the patient.

Oesophageal reflux

Reflux oesophagitis is common condition, occurring at any age, caused by transient or persistent loss of tone of the lower oesophageal sphincter.

Reflux oesophagitis causes a retrosternal burning sensation, described by the patient as heartburn.

If the oesophagus becomes very inflamed the patient will also have dysphagia.

Bending, stooping, heavy lifting and tight clothes all force acid up into the oesophagus and cause heartburn.

Oesophageal reflux can be demonstrated in 30-40% of the population.

Clinical Features

These include:

- Retrosternal or epigastric pain described by the patient as heartburn or a burning sensation:
  - aggravated by postural change such as bending, stooping, or lying down, and by tight clothing which forces acid up into the oesophagus.
  - may be referred to the neck, shoulder or arms, so mimicking angina.
- Reflux is bitter or sour, reflecting its origin from the stomach. It is relieved by alkali.
- Dysphagia—a late symptom. It may be caused by muscle spasm secondary to irritation, or be due to oedema, inflammation, spasm or rarely, stricture resulting from acid peptic regurgitation.
- "Globus hystericus"—a chronic sensation of a foreign object lodged in the throat, tightness of the throat and a difficulty to initiate swallowing. Believed to be due to irritation and spasm in the cricopharyngeal sphincter region.

- Respiratory symptoms—recurrent pneumonia, lung abscess and bronchiectasis—but a causal relationship is unproven. Coarse crepitations may be discernible at the lung bases.
- Pallor due to occult bleeding and consequent anaemia and lethargy.
- Haematemesis—due to ulcerative bleeding.
- Odynophagia.

Reflux oesophagitis is due to gastro-oesophageal reflux.

Differential Diagnosis

- Angina pectoris
- Chronic cholecystitis
- Peptic ulcer.

Dyspepsia Guidelines

Perform ELISA blood test for Helicobacter pylori antibody:

- All H.pylori positive patients should receive a course of triple therapy.
- Patients under 45 with no alarm symptoms or signs:
  - Try anti-secretory(ulcer-healing) treatment for 2-4 weeks.
  - If no evidence of H.pylori or there are no symptoms after treatment, gastroscopy is not recommended.
  - If H.pylori positive and symptoms persist after treatment, refer for gastroscopy.
- Patients under 45 with alarm symptoms or signs
  - Refer for gastroscopy
- All patients over 45:
  - Refer for gastroscopy and biopsy at the first onset of persistent dyspepsia (new onset dyspepsia).
  - Anti-secretary treatment for 2-4 weeks may be acceptable before investigation if gastroscopy cannot be provided promptly.

Investigations

If the patient suffers from heartburn then no investigation is needed providing that there is response to measures such as weight reduction, dietary advice and anti-acids, and the patient is under 40 years of age.

If heartburn does not respond to these measures, becomes more frequent, or the patient is older than 40 years, then investigation is required.

The first line investigation is upper GI endoscopy. This is the most sensitive means of diagnosing oesophagitis. However, in about 30% of patients with symptomatic gastro-oesophageal reflux there is no endoscopic abnormality. If the endoscopy confirms oesophagitis and excludes other pathologies then this gives a firm diagnosis. If the endoscopy reveals no abnormality but the symptoms are characteristic of reflux oesophagitis then medical treatment may still be initiated without further investigation.

If the symptoms are not characteristic of oesophageal reflux, or the response to medical treatment is inadequate, then 24-hour pH monitoring is indicated. A positive diagnosis of reflux oesophagitis is made if there is a pH of less than 4 for more than 5% of the time which correspond to episodes of heartburn.

Management of Reflux Oesophagitis

General first-line measures against reflux oesophagitis include:

- Losing weight
- Stopping smoking
- Elevating the head of the bed
- Not lying down before a meal
- Not eating before bedtime
- Reducing the size of meals proton pump inhibitors in gastro-oesophageal reflux disease
- A healing dose of a proton pump inhibitor (PPI) should be prescribed in patients with severe symptoms of gastro-oesophageal reflux disorder

(GORD) or who have proven pathology (1) (oesophageal ulceration or Barrett's oesophagus).

- After symptomatic control has been achieved then the dose should be reduced to the lowest dose that allows symptomatic control.
- The higher healing dose should be recommenced if there is a recurrence of GORD symptoms.
- In cases of complicated oesophagitis (e.g. haemorrhage, stricture) the the higher healing dose should be maintained.
- In patients who do not have proven pathology/mild symptoms of GORD then often alternative therapies to PPIs can be used in management e.g. alginates, antacids, H2 receptor antagonists.
- In severe cases a H2-antagonist may be used in addition
- In some patients, gastric motility stimulants may be effective, by increasing the rate of gastric emptying and hence, reducing the opportunity for reflux. Metoclopramide and domperidone, may be of use in stimulation of gastric emptying, particularly in patients with systemic sclerosis, diabetes mellitus, and autonomic neuropathy. Cisapride has been withdrawn from marketing in the UK (2).

The treatment of reflux oesophagitis with omeprazole in patients who are *H. pylori* positive increases the risk of atrophic gastritis (3).

If the condition is intractable then surgical intervention may be indicated. This amounts to 5% of patients seen by a specialist, usually people troubled by the volume of fluid regurgitated rather than by the oesophagitis. The operation of choice is fundoplication which may be carried out in an open manner via transthoracic or transabdominal approaches, or via a laparoscope.

Oesophageal Perforation

Perforation or rupture of the oesophagus is an important differential diagnosis in chest pain. Clinically, pain follows vomiting and a chest radiograph shows left pleural effusion with gas in the mediastinum. There may be distress, dysphagia and dyspnoea.

It should not be confused with Mallory-Weiss tear, which is a tear in the mucosa of the oesophagus, and thus, is managed more conservatively.

Aetiology

Possible causes of oesophageal perforation include:

- Iatrogenic:
  - endoscopy
  - gastroscopy
  - surgery.
- Non-iatrogenic:
  - caustic ingestion
  - trauma e.g. knife wound
  - foreign body
  - carcinoma
  - varices
  - diverticulitis.
  - spontaneous perforation—Boerhaave's syndrome.

Clinical Features

After instrumentation, perforation of the oesophagus is suspected if the patient complains of pain in the neck, chest or upper abdomen, together with dysphagia and pyrexia; this may not be evident immediately if the patient is sedated.

The sedated patient may suddenly become cyanosed and tachycardic. Surgical emphysema felt in the supraclavicular area supports the diagnosis.

Spontaneous rupture of the oesophagus is rare; it is associated with violent vomiting after a large meal. The patient has severe chest pain, and pain in the dorsal region of the spine or the upper abdomen. The patient is collapsed and cyanosed; the abdomen may be rigid and often a false diagnosis of perforated peptic ulcer is made.

Treatment

The important features are:

- Prompt recognition.
- Nil by mouth until at least the fifth day after diagnosis; oral feeding is withheld until a contrast swallow confirms healing at this stage.
- Pleural space drained.
- Hyperalimentation with hypertonic glucose and amino acids; this allows infection to be more readily controlled and encourages wound healing.
- Antibiotics e.g. combination of intravenous gentamicin, cefuroxime and metronidazole.
- Fluid resuscitation.
- Surgical repair if recognised early. If there is a late presentation then surgical drainage and diversion may be needed.

Oesophageal Varices

Oesophageal varices are varicosities of branches of the azygos vein which anastomose with tributaries of the portal vein in the lower oesophagus, due to portal hypertension in conditions such as cirrhosis of the liver.

Only about 30% of patients with varices ever bleed. There is more likelihood of bleeding with increasing size of the varicosities.

Aetiology

Oesophageal varices result from portal hypertension. Less than one fifth of the normal portal circulation passes through the liver due to increased resistance to flow. Hence, the majority of the splanchnic blood flow must find alternative routes back to the heart: there are several collateral channels, e.g. the middle and inferior rectal veins. However, the most important pass via the large submucous varices protruding into the lumen in the upper part of the stomach and lower end of the oesophagus. These drain the coronary vein of the stomach into the azygous and hemiazygous parts of the systemic circulation.

Clinical Features

Varices may remain asymptomatic.

The commonest presentation of symptomatic varices is brisk haematemesis. If the varices bleed slowly then the patient may present with melaena or anaemia. In many patients the stigmata of chronic liver disease, e.g. liver palms, spider naevi, ecchymoses, may be present. Large varices bleed and these usually accompany portal pressures of greater than 14mm Hg.

Investigation

Investigation of suspected oesophageal varices involves endoscopy which permits identification of the site of bleeding as well as enabling treatment, e.g. endoscopic sclerotherapy.

Angiography is used in specialist centres to delineate the varices and the cause of portal hypertension.

Management of Bleeding Oesophageal Varices

Initial resuscitation of the patient:

- IV access and cross-match blood
- Test for hypoglycaemia
- CVP line
- Consider Swan-Ganz catheter in those with ascites or associated medical problem
- Transfuse colloid, then cross matched whole blood

After initial resucitation then early endoscopy, optimally within four hours, enables accurate identification of the bleeding site, which may not always be from varices.

Measures are employed to halt the bleeding:

- If endoscopic expertise is available then:
  - if oesophageal varices, then injection sclerotherapy or band ligation
  - if gastric varices, then alternatives include injection sclerotherapy, tissue adhesives or thrombin.

- If unsuccessful or as an adjunct to endoscopic treatment then a vasoactive agent may be given—evidence suggests that combination of somatostatin or octreotide and endoscopic therapy is more effective than either alone in controlling an initial oesophageal variceal bleed (1).
- If bleeding persists then balloon tamponade with a Sengstaken-Blakemore tube should be considered.
- Other measures include:
  - transjugular intrahepatic portal-systemic stent shunt
  - oesophageal transection with anastomosis
  - variceal transthoracic transoesophageal ligation
  - Tanner operation—involves gastric transection with reanastomosis.

Plummer-Vinson Syndrome

Plummer Vinson syndrome is the formation of an oesophageal web above the aortic arch in association with concomitant iron deficiency in women.

Sometimes there may be chronic atrophic glossitis, koilonychia, angular stomatitis and achlorhydria. The main complaint is of dysphagia.

The condition is premalignant and is associated with the development of a carcinoma in the cricopharyngeal region. Initial treatment is by balloon dilatation at endoscopy and iron replacement medication. Once anaemia is corrected and a fuller diet can be taken orally, there is dramatic symptomatic improvement.

It is the only head and neck malignant condition occurring more often in women than in men. The developing carcinoma is radiosensitive.

STOMACH DISEASES AND CONDITIONS

Bezoars

A bezoar is a mass of swallowed foreign material within the stomach. The material may be hair—a trichobezoar—vegetable elements such as leaves—a phytobezoar, or other unusual items. They are usually ingested by psychiatrically disturbed patients or are a result of delayed gastric emptying, for example after gastric surgery.

The mass of material may fill the whole of the stomach. This results in the symptoms of obstruction and ulceration with subsequent disrupted nutrition and loss of weight.

Treatment is ideally removal of the bezoar endoscopically, but laparotomy and gastrotomy may be required. Phytobezoars have been treated with oral cellulase enzyme, such as 75 mg in solution with food.

Gastric Ulcer

Gastric ulcers occur three times more commonly in males than in females, with the highest incidence between ages 40 and 80 years.

There is some evidence that at least some gastric ulcers are due to an excess of the antral hormone, gastrin; thus they may be cured by antrectomy in which the gastric ulcer itself is left *in situ*.

They may complicate pyloric stenosis where food stasis stimulates prolonged antral secretion of gastrin.

Epidemiology of Gastric Ulcer

- Common condition in late middle age—incidence increases with age.
- Approximately twice as common in males than in females.
- More common in patients with blood group A.
- Was more common in lower socio-economic groups—this seems to be changing.
- Use of NSAIDs—associated with a three- to four-fold increase in risk of gastric ulcer.
- Less related to Helicobacter pylori than duodenal ulcers—*H. pylori* can be isolated from 70% of patients with gastric ulcers compared to over 95% of patients with duodenal ulcers.

Clinical Features of a Gastric Ulcer

The Clinical Features of a gastric ulcer include:

- Epigastric discomfort or pain:
  - may vary from a vague and mild discomfort, which is ignored, to a very severe pain that makes the patient lie down
  - the pain occurs 15 to 30 minutes after eating
  - the pain is relieved by vomiting and made worse by eating—thus these patients often complain of weight loss rather than the weight gain associated with duodenal ulcers—the patient may complain of being 'afraid to eat'
  - pain often worst during the day; pain is often worst during the night in duodenal ulceration
  - pain lasts for a period of about 2 weeks and occurs in cycles of every 1-2 months.
- Acidbrash, waterbrash and heartburn are symptoms common to both types of ulcer, but occur slightly more often in patients with duodenal ulcers.
- Haematemesis and melaena may complicate all forms of peptic ulceration examination is likely to be normal. There is usually no more than mild to *investigations.*
- A suspected gastric ulcer may be a malignancy and should always be biopsied. If the lesion is identified on a barium meal then biopsies must follow. A further endoscopy must occur after treatment to ensure healing. Most benign gastric ulcers occur on the lesser curve of the stomach or in the prepyloric region.
- Duodenal ulceration is almost never the site of malignancy and therefore it usually not necessary to undertake biopsies. In this case, diagnosis can be be made on barium meal or endoscopy. A follow-up endoscopy to ensure healing after treatment if the patient has become asymptomatic is generally not required.

- Gastrin levels if suspected Zollinger-Ellinson syndrome—numerous or difficult to treat ulcers.
- Acid-output studies are not often required.
- Tests for H.pylori are now considered to be very important.
- Moderate epigastric tenderness.

Treatment

Medical treatment of a gastric ulcer entails advice about:

- Discouraging smoking.
- Not avoiding spicy foods, coffee or alcohol unless these foodstuffs cause exacerbation of symptoms.

H_2-receptor antagonists are the usual first choice medical treatment in this condition, e.g. cimetidine or ranitidine.

Specific Points: Medical Management of Gastric Ulcer

- Ideally a gastroscopy should be performed with a biopsy and cytology for every patient with a gastric ulcer.
- *H. pylori* eradication therapy (triple therapy) is indicated because 70% of gastric ulcers are *H. pylori* positive.
- The British Society of Gastroenterology guidelines on the management of dyspepsia advise a further two months' antisecretory therapy since gastric ulcers take longer to heal after eradication alone; *H. pylori* negative gastric ulcers require 8 weeks antisecretory therapy with if possible, withdrawal of NSAIDs—the authors of the BSG report suggest that treatment with a proton pump inhibitor is more effective if the NSAID has to be continued.
- Follow-up
  - Repeat endoscopy with biopsies is essential until complete epithelialisation in all cases of gastric ulcer. If the ulcer remains unhealed for six months then consider surgery.

Surgical Management

Indicated if there is either:

- Failure of medical treatment
- Complications, e.g. recurrent haemorrhage, perforation, outflow obstruction
- A possibility of malignancy.

Different operations that may be performed include:

- Vagotomy
- Partial gastrectomy.

Complications:

- Post-parandial hypoglycaemia (late dumping), dizziness and lethargy soon after eating may follow a vagotomy.
- Dizziness and lethargy soon after eating due to the osmotic effect of large volumes of food in the proximal small intestine (early dumping).
- Ulcer relapse—more common after a highly selective vagotomy than a truncal vagotomy.

Gastric Volvulus

Gastric volvulus—the torsion of the stomach—may be mesenteroaxial, i.e. vertically-disposed, or organoaxial, i.e. horizontally. Most commonly, the colon shifts upwards under the diaphragm, often into an hiatal defect, and takes the stomach with it.

Clinically, it usually presents with nausea, vomiting, and retching, and it is noted on investigation that a nasogastric tube will not pass into the stomach. A chronic form may present more insidiously. Diagnosis is made by barium enema.

Emergency surgery is required if spontaneous reduction does not occur rapidly. The concern is that ischaemia will lead to gangrene and perforation. The greater curve of the stomach is freed from its colonic attachment. The risk of recurrence may be minimised by fixing the stomach, e.g. to the duodenojejunal flexure.

Gastrocolic Fistula

A gastrocolic fistula is a passage between gastric epithelium and epithelium of the colon. It may be a complication of a gastric ulcer or gastroenterostomy procedure.

This condition may cause diarrhoea, weight loss, belching of fetid gas or, very rarely, vomiting of faeculant material.

Diagnosis is made primarily on the history. Barium enema may miss the majority of fistulas.

Treatment entails resection of the fistula, possibly combined with partial gastrectomy. Supportive measures must also be taken: the individual is often malnourished.

Menetrier's Disease

Menetrier's disease is a disease of the stomach characterised by giant hypertrophy of the mucosa of the gastric fundus with cystic changes in the crypts; the antrum is spared. It is associated with protein loss—sometimes to the point of peripheral oedema. It is treated by partial gastrectomy, although the subsequent likelihood of malnutrition due to surgery must be weighed against the present nutritional deficit.

It may predispose to malignancy— stomach carcinoma developed in 10% of cases.

The condition should be distinguished from hyper-rugosity of the gastric mucosa in which there is no protein loss and which may be associated with the Zollinger-Ellison syndrome.

Pyloric Stenosis

Pyloric stenosis is a condition where the pylorus of the stomach is stenosed, and will thus not allow the passage of food.

Pyloric Stenosis (infantile)

SEE IN THE PAEDIATRIC SURGERY SECTION

Pyloric Stenosis (adult)

An adult with pyloric stenosis presents with vomiting which is usually large in volume, not bile-stained and, if the condition is long-standing, not acidic because gastric acid secretion is reduced.

The stomach contents are not digested and the patient may recognize food that was eaten 24 or 48 hours previously. Apart from the epigastric distension, visible gastric peristalsis *aetiology*

Adult pyloric stenosis occurs most commonly as a result of peptic ulceration, where at first fibrotic scarring is compensated by dilatation and hypertrophy of the stomach muscle. The process of compensation eventually fails to keep pace—similar to the failure of a hypertrophic ventricle to pump through a stenosed valve. This sort of obstruction is not specific to the pylorus.

Other causes of pyloric stenois include:

- Tumour, e.g. cancer of the stomach, commonly, carcinoma of the antrum; rarely, Hodgkin's disease
- Vagotomy, used in the treatment of intractable gastric ulceration. A pyloroplasty is performed in an effort to prevent this and a succussion splash, there may be no other abnormal physical signs.

Clinical Features

The Clinical Features of adult pyloric stenosis include:

- Characteristic profuse vomiting, free from bile, but may contain food eaten one or two days previously
- Copious vomiting may cause associated:
  - Loss of weight
  - Constipation—because of dehydration
  - Weakness due to electrolyte disturbance.

On examination, the patient may appear dehydrated and wasted. The progressive dilatation and hypertrophy of the stomach can be summed up as 'the stomach you can hear, the stomach you can hear and see, and the stomach you can hear, see and feel'.

At first a gastric splash can be elicited by shaking the patient's abdomen several hours after a meal; as the stomach enlarges, visible peristalsis also can be seen, passing from left to right across the upper abdomen. Finally, the grossly dilated, hypertrophied stomach—full of stale food and fluid, can actually be palpated.

Biochemical Disturbances

Biochemical disturbances in adult pyloric stenosis may be summarised as follows:

- The patient is dehydrated and the haematocrit level is raised.
- The urine is scanty, concentrated, initially alkaline, but later acid; its chloride content is reduced or absent.
- Serum chloride is lowered because of the vomitus losses.
- Serum sodium and potassium are lowered as a result of the kidney exchanging sodium ions and some potassium ions for hydrogen ions lost in the vomitus.
- The plasma bicarbonate is raised.
- The urea level is raised because of dehydration
- The result of all these changes is the development of a hypochloraemic alkalosis.

Diagnosis

The diagnosis of pyloric stenosis is made on the history combined with plain abdominal X-ray. It may be possible to see a grossly dilated stomach filled with mottled shadowing caused by residual food.

Radiology is supplemented by endoscopy. It is necessary to clear the gastric residue using several washouts before endoscopy or a barium meal can be attempted. More than 500ml of gastric residue may be found on nasogastric intubation.

Note that it is important for the stomach to be cleared for surgery as well as these investigative procedures.

Management

The first aim in management of adult pyloric stenosis is resuscitation of the patient. This involves correcting any electrolyte imbalances that have occurred as the result of persistent vomiting. Note that the urea will normally fall as a result of rehydration and that this intervention may unmask a chronic anaemia. The latter may require blood transfusion.

Food residues must be removed from the stomach. This may take several days administration of weak bicarbonate solution into the stomach via a large bore oesophageal tube. H2-antagonists or a proton pump inhibitor are also given at this stage to reduce any inflammatory process.

The corrective treatment of adult pyloric stenosis is surgical. There are several options but an often used technique is a truncal vagotomy with a pyloroplasty or gastroenterostomy. Proximal gastric vagotomy and stricture dilatation has also been attempted

Pyloric Hypertrophy (adult)

Adult pyloric hypertrophy is rare. There is the typical hypertrophied pyloric thickening as seen in infants and there may be a long history of gastric symptoms leading to frank pyloric obstruction. The key differential diagnoses are those of pyloric carcinoma and pyloric stenosis.

The congenital pyloric hypertrophy may have persisted and only become manifest in adult life. Treatment entails pyloroplasty or gastrojejunostomy.

SMALL INTESTINAL DISEASES AND CONDITIONS

Duodenal atresia

Duodenal atresia may be due to a complete absence of the duodenum, a fibrous band, a diaphragm, or a partial diaphragm. It most commonly occurs at the point of junction of fore- and midgut. This condition results in bile-stained vomiting.

Clinical Features

With congenital duodenal atresia, the common bile duct usually enters proximal to the obstruction and the vomit therefore usually contains bile.

Profuse vomiting occurs from birth and the stomach may be visibly distended.

There is an association with Down's syndrome.

Embryology

The duodenum is filled with epithelial cells at about five weeks gestation. It then undergoes vacuolization and recanalisation by week eight.

Failure of this process results in atresia.

Differential Diagnosis

- Oesophageal atresia—the baby presents with choking rather than vomiting.
- Pyloric stenosis—bile is absent from the vomitus; there is a generally palpable pyloric 'tumour'; onset is later (3-4 weeks) than duodenal atresia (at birth).
- Congenital intestinal obstruction: there is abdominal distension; abdominal X-ray reveals features of obstruction.

Plain radiography of the abdomen is diagnostic and shows distension of the stomach and proximal duodenum with the absence of gas in the rest of the bowel.

Investigations and Treatment

Duodenal atresia should be investigated by:

- Electrolyte and acid-base status measures, e.g. U and E's, blood gases, with subsequent correction of abnormalities.
- Plain abdominal X-ray: this may show a 'double bubble' sign of duodenal obstruction.
- Barium study may show stenosis.

Treatment involves surgical correction via a duodenojejunostomy with resection of the atretic section.

Associations

Duodenal atresia may be associated with Down's syndrome; the association is common enough to indicate a chromosome check on all babies with this condition.

Duodenal Ulcer

Duodenal ulcer—a break in the mucosal lining of the duodenum—is a form of peptic ulcer more prevalent in men than women with the greatest incidence in the 20 to 60 year age group.

Duodenal ulcers are about four times as common as gastric ulcers. There is a strong association between duodenal ulceration and *Helicobacter pylori* with over 95% of patients with a duodenal ulcer infected with *Helicobacter pylori*.

Epidemiology of Duodenal ulcer

- four times more common in men than women
- most common in middle age—peak 30-50 years
- strong genetic influence:
  - three times more common in first degree relatives of patients with an ulcer than in the general population
  - more common in patients with blood group O
  - more common in non-secretors of ABO blood group antigens into body fluids such as saliva

  - increased incidence in white males with HLA-B5 antigen
  - associated with increased serum pepsinogen.
- Reportedly lower incidence in lower socio-economic groups.
- *Helicobacter pylori* infection is often seen—over 95% of patients with a duodenal ulcer are infected with *H. pylori.*
- Smoking is twice as common in patients with chronic peptic ulceration than the general population.

Clinical features of a duodenal ulcer

- Pain—epigastric; radiates to the back; often worse at night.
- Onset 2 to 3 hours after eating.
- Relieved by eating and drinking milk.
- Precipitating factors include missing a meal, anxiety or stress.
- Nocturnal pain is a feature of duodenal ulceration

The pain may occur in 4 to 6 month cycles and last for 1 to 2 months.

Patients may gain weight as a result of an increased intake of food and milk. These feature are contrasted with those of gastric ulcers where the patient may become 'afraid to eat' because of the pain and loses weight because of lowered calorific intake.

Haematemesis and melaena may complicate all types of peptic ulceration.

A succussion splash this may occur in patients with gastric outlet obstruction, e.g. gastric carcinoma, chronic duodenal ulcer.

Investigations

- A suspected gastric ulcer may be a malignancy and should always be biopsied. If the lesion is identified on a barium meal then biopsies must follow. A further endoscopy must occur after treatment to ensure healing. Most benign gastric ulcers occur on the lesser curve of the stomach or in the prepyloric region.

- Duodenal ulceration is almost never the site of malignancy and therefore it usually not necessary to undertake biopsies. In this case, diagnosis can be be made on barium meal or endoscopy. A follow-up endoscopy to ensure healing after treatment if the patient has become asymptomatic is generally not required.
- Gastrin levels if suspected Zollinger-Ellinson syndrome—numerous or difficult to treat ulcers.
- Acid-output studies are not often required.
- Tests for H.pylori are now considered to be very important.

Medical Management

Drugs used in the medical management of peptic ulcer disease fall into three classes:

- Neutralization of acid—H_2 antagonists, e.g. ranitidine 150 mg bd or 300 mg nocte for 4-8 weeks. Ranitidine is preferred because it has fewer side effects and drug interactions than cimetidine. These drugs are effective in both gastric and duodenal ulcers. However, recurrence of duodenal ulcer is common once treatment is stopped, possibly because of the continued existence of *H. pylori*.
- Inhibition of acid secretion—(e.g. omeprazole) is used in the short-term for patients who have failed to respond to maximal doses of H2 antagonists, particularly in the Zollinger-Ellison syndrome.
- Increased mucosal resistance:
  - sucralfate—there is some concern about long-term use because of the drug's aluminium content. It may also reduce phenytoin absorption.
  - misoprostol—used to prevent gastric ulceration in patients taking non-steroidal anti-inflammatory drugs.

In patients with a proven duodenal or gastric ulcer, the British Society of Gastroenterology advise *H. pylori* eradication therapy (triple therapy) because of the high prevalence of *H. pylori* in patients with these conditions (duodenal ulcer—95% patients *H. pylori* positive; gastric ulcer—70% *H. pylori* positive).

Some patients may require maintenance therapy for the rest of their lives:

Surgical Treatment

Surgical treatment of simple duodenal ulceration which is resistant to medical therapy includes:

- Vagotomy and drainage
- Polya gastrectomy.

Complications

- Perforation
- GI haemorrhage
  - haematemesis and melaena, or
  - chronic slow oozing—patient with history of duodenal ulcer, tiredness, anaemic.
- *Stricture:* chronic fibrosis may eventually cause gastric outlet obstruction.

Note that if an ulcer is the anterior portion of the duodenum then it is more likely to perforate—it is more common for duodenal ulcers to perforate than gastric ulcers, which are frequently posterior.

Perforated Duodenal Ulcer

Perforated peptic ulcer occurs in men more the women and has its highest incidence in the 40 to 60 year age groups.

If a peptic ulcer erodes the wall of the stomach or duodenum at a point where it is covered by visceral peritoneum, the lumen of the gut becomes connected to the peritoneal cavity. Subsequent escape of gastric acid or alkaline bile into the peritoneal cavity causes a chemical and later a bacterial peritonitis which is acutely painful.

The majority of patients give a history of indigestion or epigastric pain typical of a duodenal or gastric ulcer.

It is important to enquire whether the patient has taken any steroids or aspirin because both of these drugs can cause ulcers and exacerbate old ulcers to the point of perforation.

Clinical Features of Perforated Peptic Ulcer

Perforated peptic ulcer is characterised by severe, constant, sudden onset epigastric pain that often requires high doses of opiate analgesia before the patient settles. There may be haematemsis.

On examination:

- Patient looks ill and lies unusually still
- In pain
- Tachycardia
- Shallow respiration

Inspection:

- Abdomen is flat—does not fall and rise with respiration

Palpation:

- Very tender, intense guarding & "board-like" rigidity.

Percussion:

- If air has escaped into the peritoneal cavity then the liver dullness may be absent.

Auscultation:

- Bowel sounds do not disappear until 6 to 12 hours after the onset of pain.

Peptic ulcer perforation results in a chemical peritonitis rather than a bacterial peritonitis in the initial stages—unlike perforations of the more distal bowel. Thus, in the first 24 hours or so, the patient does not show signs of general toxicity. After this period secondary bacterial infection occurs and signs of sepsis are present.

Note that if a posterior gastric ulcer perforates then the gastric contents leak into the lesser sac. This condition presents more insidiously than other peptic ulcer perforations.

Epidemiology

Perforated peptic ulcer occurs in men more then women and has its highest incidence in the 40 to 60 year age groups.

Other epidemiological points of note:

- Often associated with NSAIDs or steroid treatment in patients with peptic ulcer disease.
- More rarely associated with stress such as trauma and major burns.
- Perforations of duodenal ulcers are three times more common than gastric ulcer perforations.
- Gastric ulcer perforations are:
  - uncommon
  - most common in the elderly
  - in a third due to perforation of a gastric carcinoma.
- Oesophageal peptic ulcers are a very rare cause of peptic ulcer perforation.

Investigations

The three principle conditions in the differential diagnosis of a suspected perforated peptic ulcer are acute pancreatitis, acute cholecystitis, and another perforated viscus e.g. colon diverticula. Investigations are directed at discriminating these conditions and preparing patient for possible surgery.

- Blood tests—FBC, U+Es, LFTs, amylase, group and save
- Erect CXR—may show gas under the diaphragm—and plain abdominal film
- ECG
- Gastroscopy is contraindicated: this is because the stomach is inflated during this procedure, and air and gastric contents would be propelled into the peritoneal cavity.

Management

The management of perforated peptic ulcer entails:
- Patient is made nil by mouth.
- Analgesia—i.m. pethidine.
- Antiemetic—i.m. prochlorperazine.
- Treatment is usually surgical:
  - The duodenal ulcer is oversown either at open laparotomy or laparoscopically:
    - § when perforation and bleeding occur simultaneously, a Billroth II partial gastrectomy is advisable
  - the gastric ulcer, due to its tendency in one third of cases to be malignant, and also because of an increased tendency to breakdown after repair, is usually treated with a partial gastrectomy; simple oversewing may be contemplated when the ulcer is:
    - § close to the pylorus
    - § due to steroids or stress
    - § when the patient is in extremis
- Rarely, a perforation may become walled-off by fibrin and omentum, conservative management with nasogastric suction is instituted, and the patient improves without recourse to surgery.

Prognosis

- Mortality—5-10%
- Age over 70 years carries a poor prognosis.

Crohn's disease

Crohn's disease is a disorder of unknown aetiology that is characterised pathologically by involvement of all bowel wall layers in a chronic inflammatory process with non-caseating granulomas. The granulomatous inflammation most frequently affects the terminal ileum but it may affect any part of the gastrointestinal tract and frequently affected areas are in discontinuity. There is a tendency to form fistulae.

Epidemiolology

- Prevalence is 30-50 per 100,000.
- Women more affected than men
- Most commonly affected age group is between 15 and 35 years. There is also a second peak in the elderly.
- Familial clustering and involves ulcerative colitis as well as Crohn's disease.
- More common in smokers than non-smokers (4:1).
- Most common site of disease is the terminal ileum.

Aetiology

The cause of Crohn's disease is unknown. Several factors have been suggested:

- Genetic—in up to 20% of patients with Crohn's disease there is another family member affected by Crohn's or ulcerative colitis. There is a weak association with HLA-DR1 and DRQ5 in California, USA
- Smoking—increased risk of Crohn's
- Infective organism—the following are suggestions, none are proven:
  - Mycobacterium paratuberculosis causes a granulomatous inflammation in the small intestine of cattle.
  - persistence of measles virus; those born at the time of measles epidemics seem to be at higher risk.
- Diet—low intake of fibre from fruit and vegetables has been associated with the development of Crohn's.
- Immune mechanisms—may be a down-regulating of the normal mucosal immune response in Crohn's.

Pathological Features

Macroscopically in Crohn's disease there may be a swollen, reddened and rubbery bowel with:

- Skip lesions—discontinuous sites of pathology along the gastrointestinal tract.
- Cobblestone ulceration; a result of apthous ulceration progressing to oedema and nodular thickening
- Lead pipe thickening—thickened, stiff bowel.
- Narrowed lumen.
- Strictures.
- 'Rose-thorn' narrow-mouthed ulcers which lead to fistulae.
- Fistulae, often between adherent bowel and/or bladder, vagina, other abdominal organs or the abdominal wall.
- Mesenteric fat covering serosa.
- Enlarged mesenteric nodes.

Microscopically, there is:

- Non-caseating granulomas—not always present
- Transmural inflammation and lymphocyte infiltration.

Crohn's disease may involve any part of the bowel from the mouth to the anus:

- The terminal ileum is involved in nearly 50% of cases.
- Jejunoileitis is also seen, but most ileal inflammation usually ends abruptly at the ileocaecal junction.
- Caecal and right colonic involvement is more common than lesions in the stomach and duodenum.

Clinical Features

This is a chronic, relapsing and remitting disease that has symptomatology dependent on the site of involvement of the GI tract. The commonest site at presentation is the terminal ileum and proximal colon.

Various symptoms occur in most patients:

- Abdominal pain
- Weight loss
- Diarrhoea.

Special note must be taken that:

- Crohn's disease may present with an acute onset of abdominal pain that may mimic acute appendicitis or yersinia ileitis.
- common features in active disease are lassitude, anorexia, malaise, and fever.
- in adolescents, a presentation with weight loss alone (without abdominal pain or diarrhoea) may be misdiagnosed as anorexia nervosa.

Differential Diagnosis

The differential diagnosis of Crohn's disease includes:

- Ulcerative colitis. In 10 to 20% of cases the two diseases cannot be differentiated. Distinguishing features include rectal involvement and bloody diarrhoea in UC, continuous disease pathology, but no strictures or fistulae. In UC there is a low plasma IL-6 in the active disease, and there is a stronger association with non-smokers. Also, UC patients are more often p-ANCA positive.
- *Irritable bowel syndrome.* This has no radiological abnormalities or weight loss.
- Gastrointestinal malignancy. The most important cancers here are lymphoma, right colonic cancer and small bowel cancer. These patients might be expected to have night sweats and anaemia. Radiologically there may be a mass and metastases.
- Ileal tuberculosis. This should be investigated for with a stool culture, and might be suspected in the immigrant population. Pathologically, after laparoscopic biopsy there will be caseating granulomas and mesenteric tubercules.
- Anorexia nervosa
- Coeliac disease—this will cause a malabsorptive picture.
- Chronic infection with Giardia, Yersinia and Campylobacter.
- Amyloidosis.

- Behcet's disease
- Whipple's disease.

Investigations

Investigations in Crohn's disease are aimed at:

- Making the diagnosis
- Monitoring disease activity.

To this end, a variety of modalities may be used:

- Blood tests
- Imaging
- *Endoscopy:* both upper and lower GI endoscopy.
- *Histology:* full thickness inflammation, non-caseating granulomata, fissuring, ulceration, erosions.

Diagnosis

Diagnosis of Crohn's disease is based on clinical, radiological and pathological evidence of the disease.

It involves a careful history of chronic, remitting disease—the problems may take months or years to clinically manifest, barium studies of small and large bowel showing narrowing—Kantor's string sign of the terminal ileum—and skip lesions, stool culture, sigmoidoscopy and rectal biopsy, and colonoscopy with multiple biopsy.

Crohn's disease confined to the colon may be difficult to discriminate from ulcerative colitis. Features that may help discriminate the two conditions are described under 'diagnosis of ulcerative colitis'.

Complications/Associations

The complications of Crohn's disease are best considered as local or general; the general complications include some of the extraintestinal manifestations of Crohn's disease.

Local

Possible local complications of Crohn's disease include:

- Intestinal obstruction

- Haemorrhage
- Perforation with abscess
- Stricture formation; common
- Perianal abscess fistula
- Fistulae to the bowel, bladder, vagina
- Increased risk of malignancy but less than that of ulcerative colitis.

General

Common complications include:
- Weight loss
- Anaemia
- Arthritis—large joints
- Erythema nodosum
- Ocular problems—conjunctivitis, episcleritis, iritis
- Sacroiliitis—this is unrelated to HLA B27
- Gall stones, especially of the cholesterol type.

Less common:

- Liver complications—primary sclerosing cholangitis, fatty liver, non-specific hepatitis, pericholangitis.
- Ankylosing spondylitis—related to HLA B27.
- Pyoderma gangrenosum.
- Carcinoma of the bile ducts and primary sclerosing cholangitis—much less common than in ulcerative colitis.
- Renal complications—ureteric stricture, stones, right hydronephrosis, nephropathy (oxalate, amyloid).
- Nutritional deficiency—osteomalacia, weakness (potassium, magnesium, vitamin D), lassitude (vitamin B12, folate, iron), rashes (zinc, niacin), alteration of taste (zinc).
- systemic amyloidosis—more common in Crohn's than UC.
- reduced fertility.

Management

There is no medical or surgical cure for Crohn's disease. If the symptoms are due to inflammation then they generally respond to medical measures. Surgical intervention is usually required when symptoms are due to strictures.

Medical Management of Crohn's Disease

The medical management of Crohn's disease is difficult.

The general management principles are outlined in management of inflammatory bowel disease.

Information relating to particular treatment options is also included:

- Aminosalicylates
- **Corticosteroids—used in acute disease**
- Steroid-sparing agents
- Metronidazole
- Cholestyramine
- Elemental diet
- Anti-TNF-alpha agents.

There is clear evidence that stopping smoking reduces the risk of recurrence.

Surgical Management

Surgical intervention is limited in Crohn's disease because:

- The whole alimentary tract may be affected from mouth to anus
- The disease is often active at more than one site.

Consequently, there is a high incidence of post-operative complications following surgery, and a concept of minimal surgical intervention has thus been reached.

Indications

Indications for surgery in Crohn's disease include:

- Persistent ill-health with intractable disease despite medical management.
- Retardation of physical and sexual development in children.

- Intestinal obstruction that does not respond to medical therapy.
- Toxic dilatation of the colon.
- Perforation, external fistula or abscess formation.
- Periureteric inflammation causing ureteric obstruction.
- Suspicion of carcinomatous change.

Crohn's Disease and Pregnancy

If Crohn's disease flares up during pregnancy, sulphasalazine and steroids are permitted. Azathioprine and metronidazole should be avoided unless advised by a specialist. However, note that there is no convincing proof that azathioprine has been responsible for foetal abnormalities and many inflammatory bowel disease specialists now recommend continuing the drug for those patients in whom relapse would be a major problem.

There is no predicatable pattern to inflammatory bowel disease in pregnancy. Patients with inflammatory bowel disease often seem to be healthier during pregnancy, but at a risk of a flare-up in the postpartum period.

Prognosis

- Most patients have a chronic intermittent disease course, while 13% have an unremitting disease course and 10% have a prolonged remission.
- Less than half require corticosteroids at any point.
- During any given year, approximately 10% are treated with corticosteroids and 30% are treated with 5-aminosalicylates.
- Up to 57% of patients require at least one surgical resection.
- About one tenth of patients have prolonged remission.
- Nearly 75% of patients have a chronic intermittent course, and about one eighth have an unremitting course.

- If the patient has both small and large bowel disease then about 70% will require surgical intervention.

The atypical form of Crohn's is an acute ileitis. This, unlike other forms of Crohn's, does not recur and may represent a completely different disease.

The excess mortality in patients with Crohn's disease is approximately double that of the general population. This is due to the complications of active disease.

Small Bowel Obstruction

Small bowel obstruction is primarily characterised by the early onset of vomiting followed by constipation. It is commonly due to mechanical obstruction, intrinsic or extrinsic lesions. It may be partial or complete.

Small bowel obstruction can also result from paralysis of the intestinal musculature—paralytic ileus.

Aetiology

Causes of small bowel obstruction can be divided into:

- Dynamic:
  - mechanical causes obstructing lumen:
    - § tumours
    - § intussusception
    - § gallstone ileus
    - § impacted faeces
    - § meconium
    - § bezoars.
  - intrinsic lesions of the bowel wall:
  - strictures, congenital, inflammatory, neoplastic, etc.
  - extrinsic lesions:
    - § postoperative adhesions
    - § inflammation
    - § herniae

  § neoplastic masses
  § abscesses
  § volvulus.
- Adynamic—lack of peristalsis:
  – paralytic ileus
  – mesenteric vascular occlusion.

Clinical Features of Small Bowel Obstruction

Symptoms of small bowel obstruction include:
- Abdominal pain, colicky, i.e. returns to normal periodically. Felt in mid-abdomen. Need to know site, radiation, duration and relieving factors.
- No flatus; constipation is present
- Distention, early in the course of the illness if the obstruction is high
- Vomiting, again earlier in the course if the obstruction is relatively proximal in the bowel.

Signs of obstruction include:
- General appearance: dehydration due to loss of fluid from ECF when vomiting. The gastrointestinal tract secretes 6 litres of fluid per day and during obstruction, this tends to be sequestered. Hypovolaemia may result in hypotension and tachycardia.
- Inspection and palpation may reveal scars, distension, peristalsis, hernias, but no tenderness. If the blood supply is cut off then there can be congestion, ischaemia, necrosis/gangrene and perforation; tenderness develops.
- Auscultation: hyperactive—borborygmus—or ileus.
- Rectal examination: may be empty after 24 to 48 hours of symptoms.

Investigations

Tests indicated for small bowel obstruction include:
- Blood urea and electrolytes.
- White cell count.

- Radiology:
  - supine: obstructive picture of dilated small bowel
  - sitting: multiple air/fluid levels in obstruction
  - to distguish the site:
    - § obstructed jejenum shows transverse markings running right across the bowel
    - § in the ileum the markings are absent
    - § in large bowel obstruction, the haustral markings do not go right across the bowel.

Generally, barium meal and enema are contraindicated.

Principles of Management

The history and examination are valuable in suspected gastrointestinal obstruction to identify the approximate level of blockage.

The underlying management can be summarised as 'drip and suck'. The patient is kept nil by mouth and given intravenous fluids—the volume and type of which depend on the state of hydration and electrolyte balance. A nasogastric tube is placed in small bowel obstruction or if the patient is vomiting. This minimises the risk of aspiration of gastric contents, especially during the induction of general anaesthesia if surgery is required. Pain relief is given. Antibiotic prophylaxis against sepsis should be considered.

Indications for immediate surgery include:

- Crescendo pain.
- localised peritonism, implying perforation or ischaemia.
- Complete colonic obstruction with competent ileocaecal valve and caecum dilated to greater than 8 cm.
- "Closed loop" seen radiologically.
- Obstruction occurring as a result of hernial incarceration.

If peritonism is absent, then treatment is conservative for two or three days; i.e. nil by mouth, with nasogastric tube. If the features of obstruction do not resolve, or if there is general deterioration of the patient's condition with onset of abdominal tenderness and a tachycardia, then surgery is indicated.

Large bowel obstruction caused by faecal impaction may be treated with enemas or manual removal of faeces.

Non-mechanical bowel obstruction will usually resolve with conservative treatment and removal of any precipitating cause.

Small Intestine Tumours

Tumours of the small intestine are very rare. Although this region comprises 80% of the luminal surface area of the gut, fewer than 2% of all primary gastrointestinal malignancies arise here.

Classification is as follows:

- Benign
- Hamartomatous
- Intermediate
- Malignant.

Hamartomatous Lesions

Hamartomata of the small intestine include the following conditions:

- ectopic pancreas—usually seen along the antimesenteric border of the bowel or in a Meckel's diverticulum.
- Hereditary haemorrhagic telangiectasia:
  - Osler-Weber-Rendu disease
  - associated with Turner's syndrome.
- Neurofibromas and arteriovenous malformation—likely to cause symptoms such as obstruction, bleeding and intussception.
- Peutz-Jeghers syndrome:
  - polypoid lesions mainly reside in the jejunum, but can occur at any point in the gastrointestinal tract

  - intussusception of the polyps can give rise to small bowel obstruction.

Hereditary Haemorrhagic Telangiectasia

Hereditary haemorrhagic telangiectasia is a rare autosomal dominant condition where multiple small telangiectases occur on the skin and mucous membranes, most commonly on the lips and the tongue. Lesions are also often scattered over the pulps of fingers. The size and number of lesions increases with age.

Epistaxis is the most common complaint.

When telangiectases are present in the gastrointestinal tract they may cause chronic blood loss with iron deficiency anaemia. Occasionally there may be torrential bleeding.

Arteriovenous malformations may occur in the:

- Liver
- Lungs, causing:
  - clubbing
  - murmurs
  - paradoxical emboli.

Oestrogen may be used to reduce the severity and frequency of epistaxes (via induction of metaplasia of nasal mucosa).

Embolization may be used if there are pulmonary arteriovenous malformations.

Benign Tumours

Every type of cell type within the wall of the small intestine has the potential for neoplasia. The most common are:

- Adenoma, especially in the duodenum:
  - tubular: low premalignant potential
  - villous: strong potential for malignancy
  - Brunner's gland adenoma: no potential for malignancy.
- Lipoma
- Angioma

- Leiomyoma
- Fibromyoma.

They are seldom discovered during the patient's lifetime because they are generally asymptomatic. When symptomatic, problems include ulceration and haemorrhage. Treatment is by local resection.

Intermediate

There are four types of benign small bowel tumours that have a strong tendency for malignant change. Each shows a spectrum of activity from truly benign to frank cancer. They include:

- Villous adenoma:
  - closely associated with carcinoma
  - small bowel polyps may accompany up to half of all cases of Gardner's syndrome.
- Smooth muscle tumours:
  - may present with haemorrhage, obstructive symptoms or a palpable mass
  - treated by wide resection and occasionally respond to chemotherapy.
- Duodenal apudomas:
  - 10% of all gastrinomas arise at this site
  - treated by local excision or pancreatoduodenectomy.
- Carcinoid tumours:
  - the ileum is the second most frequent site of occurrence
  - approximately one third have metastasized by the time of diagnosis.

Malignant

The key three malignant neoplasms of the small intestine are:

- Adenocarcinoma
- Lymphoma
- Secondaries from other sites.

Adenocarcinoma of the Small Intestine

The adenocarcinoma is the commonest type of malignant tumour of the small intestine. They are clustered within 25 centimetres either side of the duodenojejunal flexure; ileal carcinoma is rare except for that which is secondary to Crohn's disease.

The peak frequency of carcinoma is within the seventh decade with an equal sex distribution. The clinical presentation is one of occult bleeding and partial obstruction, or, if more proximally in the duodenum, epigastric pain, vomiting and jaundice.

Investigative measures include endoscopy with biopsy and barium studies. Treatment is by surgical resection: more proximally, a pancreaticoduodenectomy may suffice; more distally, bowel and mesenteric resection is required.

Prognosis is poor—15-25% at 5 years—mainly due to the insidious progression of the tumour.

COLONIC DISEASES AND CONDITIONS

Angiodysplasia of the Colon

Colonic angiodysplasia is a common cause of acute or chronic rectal bleeding and iron deficiency anaemia.

Angiodysplasias are tiny—1-5 mm in diameter—hamartomatous capillary lesions in the colonic wall which produce bleeding out of proportion to their size. They are believed to be acquired, possibly as a result of tension on the veins where they pass through the muscularis.

Diagnosis:

- Subtraction mesenteric arteriography may demonstrate bleeding if rapid
- Colonscopy: may visualise lesion.

Treatment:

- Electrical coagulation via the colonoscope.
- Resection of segment of colon if the above is unsuccessful.

Colonic Polyps

Colonic polyps may be single or multiple. Familial polyposis coli is a condition that is inherited in autosomal dominant manner in which there is extensive polyposis of the large bowel.

Polyps are a common finding in the colon. All polyps have malignant potential although the majority are adenomas, i.e. benign neoplasms. A polyp may have undergone malignant change but still be at an early stage, and hence is potentially curable. All polyps should be assumed to be malignant until proved otherwise.

Types of Colonic Polyp

Colonic polyps may be:

- Neoplastic:
  - adenomas—single or associated with familial polyposis syndrome
- Hamartomatous:
  - juvenile—singly and as a juvenile polyposis syndrome
  - Peutz-Jegher's—singly and as part of Peutz-Jegher's syndrome.
- Hyperplastic
- Reactive:
  - inflammatory polyps—associated with inflammatory bowel disease and ulcerative colitis more than Crohn's disease
  - lymphoid.

Diagnosis and Management

The diagnosis and management of colonic polyps consist of:

- History and examination
- Sigmoidoscopy: about half of colonic polyps are within reach of the rigid 25cm instrument. Use of a fibreoptic sigmoidoscope allow the colon to be examined as far as the splenic flexure and any polyps can be removed at the same time with a diathermy snare.

- Barium enema: will show polyps of significant size. This is the investigation of choice for polyps of the transverse and ascending colon. Note that it may not be possible to see the whole colon well—this is particularly true of the transverse colon.
- Colonoscopy; indicated if:
  - barium enema technically unsatisfactory
  - barium enema demonstrates polyps.
- Histology; vital because:
  - reveals whether the whole polyp was removed
  - reveals whether the polyp was malignant.

Colonic Tumours

Colonic tumours may be:

- Benign:
  - adenomatous polyp
  - papilloma
  - lipoma
  - neurofibroma
  - haemangioma.
- Malignant:
  - primary:
    - § carcinoma
    - § lymphosarcoma
    - § carcinoid tumour.
- Secondary:
  - invasion from adjacent tumours, e.g. stomach, bladder, uterus and ovary.

Colon Carcinoma

The symptoms of cancer of the colon differ according to the part of the colon affected and the type of tumour, but pain is common to all types. Unexplained weakness and anaemia are characteristic of right colonic carcinoma whilst a change in bowel habit feature in left colonic carcinoma.

The majority of colon cancers are found in the sigmoid colon and at the rectosigmoid junction. These cancers are usually small, annular and ulcerated. The next common site is the caecum, where the tumours tend to be bulky and papilloform.

Types of Colon Carcinoma

The types of colonic carcinoma are divided into left-sided, right-sided and transverse types.

Colon Carcinoma (on left side of colon)

Left-sided colonic carcinoma is characterised by a change in bowel habit due to obstruction. Pain is felt in the left side of the abdomen because there is commonly involvement of the sigmoid colon and the rectosigmoid junction, and there is gross blood in the stool. The carcinoma tend to be small, annular and ulcerated. It appears as a fixed filling defect with an annular "apple core" configuration on barium enema. Usually, the patient is over 40 and commonly, over 70 years of age. Men are affected slightly more than women.

The patient with left-sided colonic carcinoma may be pale due to chronic blood loss and anaemia, and may show weight loss. The left supraclavicular lymph nodes may be enlarged.

The abdomen may be distended and the caecum palpable. The liver may be enlarged due to metastases.

Masses may be felt in the left iliac fossa which may be hard and indentable because of faeces above the tumour. They will be tender if there is surrounding inflammation, and will be dull to percussion, but the abdomen will feel normal on palpation if the mass is small and lying in the paravertebral gutter. A mass may be noted anteriorly on rectal examination if the tumour is down into the pelvis.

Hyperactive bowel sounds indicate chronic intestinal obstruction. During an attack of colic, loud high-pitched continuous gurgl.

Symptoms

The symptoms of left-sided colonic carcinoma include:

- Change in bowel habit due to obstruction.
- Cycle of alternating constipation and diarrhoea: constipation from the hold-up of faeces at the site of the tumour, which then liquefies and the patient develops spurious, offensive diarrhoea.
- Lower left abdominal pain: initially, a mild abdominal colic or ache, which after some weeks or months, becomes persistent with severe colicky exacerbations.
- A lump in the left iliac fossa or localized tenderness
- Painful micturition and change in frequency indicating involvement of the bladder.
- Darkly-coloured faeces streaked with blood, often containing mucus.

Less commonly:
- Loss of weight then anorexia
- Rectal bleeding and iron deficient anaemia
- Tenesmus.

Aetiology

The cause of colorectal carcinoma is unknown except for a small proportion of cases where there is malignant change in previous polyposis coli or ulcerative colitis. However, this disease is almost unknown in third world rural communities.

Some risk factors for the development of colorectal carcinoma are:
- Pre-existing colonic polyps
- Familial polyposis coli
- Ulcerative colitis
- Crohn's disease
- Schistosomal colitis
- Family history—first-degree relatives of patients with colorectal cancer have 2-3 fold increased risk, especially if relative was diagnosed under the age of 50.
- Environment—exposure to radiation; asbestos.
- Presence of ureterocolostomy.

- Diet—high fat, high calories, low dietary calcium, low fermentable fibre.
- Genetic markers, e.g. the chromosome 2 locus of de la Chapelle and Volgelstein may define a subset of colorectal cancer patients—hereditary non-polyposis colon cancer—that constitute about 5% of all colorectal carcinomas.

Other possible factors:

- Previous cholecystectomy—by increased presentation of bile acids to colonic bacteria for conversion into potential carcinogens.
- Previous gastric surgery for benign peptic ulcer.

Treatment

The treatment of left-sided colonic cancer is by surgery, when feasible. The aim is to resect the colon. The patient must be warned of the possibility of a permanent colostomy if the growth is unresectable or resectable and on the left-hand side. A temporary colostomy is sometimes necessary in order to protect an anastomosis made under difficult conditions.

The patient is admitted 2-3 days before the operation in order to prepare the bowel. The colon is cleared of exogenous material using laxatives and/or enemas, and cleansed of infective organisms using broad spectrum, poorly-absorbed antibiotics such as neomycin.

Usually, a left hemicolectomy or a Paul-Mickulicz procedure is performed. If the growth cannot be resected, a Hartmann's procedure is performed and a permanent colostomy created.

Colon Carcinoma (on right side of colon)

Right-sided colonic cancer implies carcinoma in the caecum, and the ascending and proximal transverse colon.

The patient usually presents with unexplained pain in the right iliac fossa plus or minus general symptoms such as anaemia, malaise and weakness. Abdominal pain often develops late in the disease because the tumour may remain silent until it has grown a considerable size.

In general, patients are over 40 years of age, and commonly the condition is seen in 70-80 year olds. Women are more affected than men.

Aetiology

The cause of colorectal carcinoma is unknown except for a small proportion of cases where there is malignant change in previous polyposis coli or ulcerative colitis. However, this disease is almost unknown in third world rural communities.

Some risk factors for the development of colorectal carcinoma are:

- Pre-existing colonic polyps.
- Familial polyposis coli.
- Ulcerative colitis.
- Crohn's disease.
- Schistosomal colitis.
- Family history—first-degree relatives of patients with colorectal cancer have 2-3 fold increased risk, especially if relative was diagnosed under the age of 50.
- Environment—exposure to radiation; asbestos
- Presence of ureterocolostomy.
- Diet—high fat, high calories, low dietary calcium, low fermentable fibre.
- Genetic markers, e.g. the chromosome 2 locus of de la Chapelle and Volgelstein may define a subset of colorectal cancer patients—hereditary non-polyposis colon cancer—that constitute about 5% of all colorectal carcinomas.

Other possible factors:

- Previous cholecystectomy—by increased presentation of bile acids to colonic bacteria for conversion into potential carcinogens.
- Previous gastric surgery for benign peptic ulcer.

Symptoms

Possible symptoms of right-sided colonic carcinoma include:

- Pallor, debility, breathlessness—due to iron deficiency anaemia caused by prolonged bleeding.
- Loss of weight and anorexia.
- Occult blood in faeces.
- Persistent, dull ache in right iliac fossa, often postprandial and mistakenly attributed to gallbladder or gastroduodenal disease. This is a late symptom.

Less commonly:

- Intestinal colic and intestinal obstruction if the growth occludes the ileocaecal valve.
- Acute appendicitis if the tumour blocks the mouth of the appendix, causing it to dilate.
- Change in bowel habit, either constipation or diarrhoea but not both alternately.

Signs

The patient with a right-sided colonic carcinoma may be pale and thin, possibly jaundiced.

The supraclavicular nodes may be palpable.

The abdomen may be generally distended or 'full' in the right iliac fossa. The right iliac fossa is often tender with some guarding of the covering muscles. A firm irregular mass may be felt which may be fixed or freely mobile. When it is mobile it tends to slip upwards into the paravertebral gutter or medially and downwards into the pelvis. It is dull to percussion.

The liver may be palpable and irregular.

The bowel sounds should be normal. Hyperactivity indicates obstruction of the ileo-caecal valve.

The faeces may contain blood.

Spread

The spread of colonic cancer is variably:

- Lymphatic:
  - most common

- through mesenteric and para-aortic nodes, and eventually, the thoracic duct
- may involve supraclavicular nodes in late stages.

- Direct extension:
  - through the bowel wall into adjacent structures, e.g. small intestine, stomach, duodenum, ureter, bladder, uterus, abdominal wall.
- Haematogenous spread:
  - 10-15% of cases
  - to liver in 75%, lung, or bone.
- Transcoelomic spread:
  - through the serosa and tumour cells into the peritoneal cavity forming local deposits of malignant nodules
  - the recto-vesical or recto-uterine pouches are often involved and on digital rectal examination can be felt as a hard shelf—Plummer's shelf
  - other common sites include omentum, and ovaries—Krukenberg tumour.
- Intraluminal metastasis:
  - exfoliated cells may become trapped in an anastomotic suture or staple line during operation "anastomotic recurrence.

Investigations

The preferred investigations for rectal carcinoma are:

- Full blood count.
- Blood film: test for iron-deficiency anaemia.
- Rectal examination: palpable mass in less than 50% of cases.
- Rigid sigmoidoscopy and proctoscopy: performed at the initial consultation—reveals tumours in sigmoid region and enables positive evidence by biopsy to be obtained.
- Flexible sigmoidoscopy.
- Stool sample: test for occult blood.
- *Colonoscopy:* enables inspection and biopsy of the higher reaches of the colon. Gives high sensitivity

if used by an experienced operator. Requires a full bowel preparation.

- Barium enema: usually reveals the tumour as a stricture or filling defect. But negative results are not uncommon, so if this occurs when the condition is suspected, repeat the investigations after a few weeks.
- *IVU:* a useful preoperative investigation if there is a risk of ureteric involvement.

A barium enema and other invasive tests can be particularly distressing and should not be undertaken lightly.

Differential Diagnosis

An initial erroneous diagnosis of colonic carcinoma is made in as many as 25% of patients once gastrointestinal symptoms appear.

Diseases producing similar local symptoms:

- Diverticular disease
- Ulcerative colitis
- Crohn's disease
- Ischaemic colitis
- Amoebiasis.

Diseases producing similar general manifestations:

- Carcinoma of stomach
- Carcinoma of pancreas
- Uraemia
- Pernicious anaemia.

Treatment

Right-sided colonic carcinoma is treated surgically, if at all feasible. The aim is to resect the affected segment of bowel.

The patient is admitted 2-3 days before the operation in order to prepare the bowel. The colon is cleared of exogenous material using laxatives and/or enemas, and cleansed of infective organisms using broad spectrum, poorly absorbed antibiotics such as neomycin.

Care is taken to look for metastases. Liver function tests, a liver scan, chest X-ray, and barium enema are valuable pre-operative investigations. Evidence of metastasis may not prevent planned surgery. Blood transfusion may be necessary if the anaemia is severe.

The terminal ileum, ascending colon and hepatic flexure are removed by right hemicolectomy. The patient can usually resume normal activities after 6 weeks.

Prognosis

The staging of colonic carcinoma is the most important determinant of survival rate and is normally expressed via Dukes classification. The overall 5 year survival rate is 35%:

- Operation for cure can be performed on about 70% of patients:
  - 10% of lesions not resectable at operation
  - 20% have liver or other distant metastases.
- Operative mortality rate is 2-6%
- 5 year survival rate for curative resection is 55%.

Complications such as obstruction or perforation adversely affect survival. Patients should be followed for recurrent, metastatic, or metachronous lesions. Faecal occult blood should be tested every 6-12 months and colonoscopy performed 1 year after operation. Surgical resection for recurrent lesions should be considered.

Once colorectal cancer has metastasised, the average survival duration without chemotherapy is 3-9 months (1). Systemic chemotherapy is rarely curative in patients with metastatic colorectal cancer except, sometimes, where metastatic disease is confined to the liver and potentially resectable after chemotherapy.

Colon Carcinoma (Transverse)

The patient with carcinoma of the transverse colon presents with a picture intermediate between that of left-sided and right-sided lesions.

A palpable mass may be noticed in the abdomen which is freely mobile in the early stages. A distended caecum indicates obstruction.

The tumour may be treated surgically by transverse colectomy.

Screening for Colon Carcinoma

Screening could potentially have a beneficial effect on outcome as only half the patients presenting with large bowel cancer have the potential for cure; earlier detection and treatment secures an improved prognosis.

Flexible sigmoidoscopy and colonoscopy are too labour-intensive, but faecal occult blood testing is a more promising technique. The 'Haemoccult' method, for example, uses guaiac resin that has been stabilised on filter paper to detect as little as 2-5 ml of blood passed per 24 hours. However, false positives can result if meat has been eaten in the last three days, and compliance with testing is often poor.

Research is targeting more sensitive and specific means of indicating occult bleeding, e.g. enzyme immunoassays, and of increasing compliance, e.g. a pad that is used to wipe the anus and is then developed. However, the debate on whether screening is cost-effective continues. Using methods that detect occult blood loss assume that all tumours bleed but this is not the case.

Treatment of Colon Cancer

Treatment of colonic carcinoma consists of wide surgical resection of the lesion.

Colorectal carcinomas are relatively unresponsive to chemotherapy but palliative chemotherapy in patients with locally advanced or metastatic disease has been shown to reduce death and progression at 12 months (1). The findings translate into a 16% absolute difference in survival and a 25% increase in progression free survival (increases in 3.7 months in median survival and 6 months in median progression free survival) in patients treated with palliative chemotherapy e.g. 5-fluorouracil alone or in combination with other chemotherapeutic agents.

The response to radiotherapy is limited by the difficulty of directing the radiation beam at the tumour without damaging surrounding structures, e.g. the bladder.

Surgical Treatment of Colon Cancer

Treatment of colonic carcinoma consists of wide surgical resection of the lesion and its regional lymphatic drainage after preparation of the bowel. The primary tumour is resected, even if distant metastases have occurred, since prevention of obstruction or bleeding may offer palliation for long periods.

The abdomen is explored to determine resectability of the tumour and to search for multiple primary carcinomas of the colon, distant metastases, and associated abdominal disease. Care is taken not to contribute to the spread of the tumour by unnecessary palpation. Some authors have even advocated occlusion of the bowel with encircling tape on either side of the lesion in order to contain exfoliated cancer cells within the segment to be resected.

The cancer-bearing portion is mobilised and removed.

Non-surgical Ttreatment of Colorectal Cancer

Colorectal carcinomas are relatively unresponsive to chemotherapy but liver metastases may occasionally be controlled by 5-fluorouracil (5 FU). At the time of the operation and for a week postoperatively, the portal vein is infused with heparin and 5 FU. This approach seems to be particularly beneficial for Dukes' C tumours.

5 FU is usually given in combination with Leucovirin. Recently other agents e.g. irinotecan, oxaliplatin have been found to also have a beneficial effect.

The response to radiotherapy is limited by the difficulty of directing the radiation beam at the tumour without damaging surrounding bowel. Also, if radiotherapy is to be useful, there must be only local invasion—sterilization of local lymph nodes will have no effect on prognosis, for example, if there is already hepatic involvement.

Raltitrexed is an inhibitor of thymidylate synthase .It is licensed for use as monotherapy when fluorouracil-based palliative therapy for colorectal cancer is inappropriate or not tolerated.

Irinotecan

Irinotecan inhibits topoisomerase-1 which catalyses the breaking and rejoining of DNA strands.

Irinotecan is licensed for first-line use in patients with advanced colorectal cancer, in combination with fluorouracil and folinic acid, and as second-line monotherapy when fluorouracil-based therapy has failed (1).

A regime of 5-fluorouracil and leucovirin and Irinotecan has been shown to be beneficial compared to a regime without Irinotecan. There was an objective response in 39% vs 21%, a longer time before tumour progression 7 months vs 4 months and a longer median survival 15 months vs 13 months (2).

Oxaliplatin

This is a diaminocyclohexane platinum compound which forms crosslinks in DNA, so inhibiting DNA replication.

Treatment with Oxaliplatin is associated with a 10% probability of an objective response when given alone or in combination with 5-fluorouracil and leucovirin in patients who have already received 5-fluoruracil.

Occult Hepatic Metastases (colorectal cancer)

Accurate preoperative staging is very important in predicting the prognosis of colorectal cancer. Significant occult hepatic metastases carry a poor prognosis. If the hepatic metastases group are subtracted from the group of apparently better-classified tumours, the prognosis of these tumours is much improved.

Intraoperative ultrasound is useful in finding occult hepatic metastases.

Prognosis

The staging of colonic carcinoma is the most important determinant of survival rate and is normally expressed via Dukes classification. The overall 5 year survival rate is 35%:

- Operation for cure can be performed on about 70% of patients:
  - 10% of lesions not resectable at operation
  - 20% have liver or other distant metastases
- Operative mortality rate is 2-6%
- 5 year survival rate for curative resection is 55%

Complications such as obstruction or perforation adversely affect survival. Patients should be followed for recurrent, metastatic, or metachronous lesions. Faecal occult blood should be tested every 6-12 months and colonoscopy performed 1 year after operation. Surgical resection for recurrent lesions should be considered.

Once colorectal cancer has metastasised, the average survival duration without chemotherapy is 3-9 months (1). Systemic chemotherapy is rarely curative in patients with metastatic colorectal cancer except, sometimes, where metastatic disease is confined to the liver and potentially resectable after chemotherapy.

Diverticular Disease

A diverticulum is an outpouching of the wall of the gut. Acquired diverticulae appear in the colon, especially the sigmoid colon, probably as a result of changes in bowel motility and the consistency of the faeces. Many believe that the condition is caused solely by the Western diet with its low roughage content.

Diverticulae are often symptomless. When they are acutely inflamed, then the condition is called diverticulitis.

This disease has a higher incidence in females and in the age group 50 to 70 years. It occurs in approximately 50% of the population over the age of 70.

Aetiology

Diverticular disease is believed to occur as a result of deficiency of dietary fibre which results in hypertrophy of both the longitudinal and circular muscle of the colon. This process of muscular hypertrophy is believed to cause hypersegmentation and lead to an increased intraluminal pressure and development of pulsion diverticulae. The evidence for this theory is scanty. Probably aging is as important a factor in the development of diverticular disease.

The sigmoid colon is most affected by diverticular disease. The condition extending for a variable distance proximally.

Diverticulae are often symptomless. However, individual diverticulae may become inflamed. This probably occurs because of obstruction of the narrow outlet of the diverticula. This causes a small diverticular abscess and inflammation—diverticulitis.

Pathology

In diverticular disease, the bowel is thickened, rigid and irregularly contracted. The diverticula never penetrate the taenia and are usually situated on the side wall between the mesenteric taenia and the two antimesenteric taenia. However, they may also arise on the antimesenteric intertaenial area.

The muscle of the bowel wall may be hypertrophied to such a degree that it seems that new growths exist—Grasser's tumour.

Clinical Features

Diverticular disease is often asymptomatic. However, all of the following may occur:

- Commonest symptom is pain or indigestion which may be very mild or severe enough to make the patient lie down.
- Persistent ache with colicky exacerbations felt in the left lower quadrant.
- No radiation.
- Not precipitated by eating.
- Distension, flatulence and belching.
- Constipation—infrequent bowel actions and hard stool.
- Appetite and weight remain normal.

On examination, there may be nothing abnormal to find, but in most patients the sigmoid colon is easily palpable and slightly tender, with tenderness throughout the whole of the left iliac fossa during an attack.

The diagnosis is made by the appearance of the bowel on barium enema.

Associated Conditions

If inflammation occurs in the diverticula, acute or chronic diverticulitis is the result.

Investigations

Diverticular disease is a diagnosis of exclusion. Hence, investigation must first rule out other treatable causes of similar symptomatology, e.g. ulcerative colitis, Crohn's disease, ischaemic colitis and colorectal carcinoma. Hence, barium meal, barium enema and sigmoidoscopy are common first-line investigations.

If acute inflammation is suspected, e.g. due to the presence of fever, leucocytosis and acute pain, these investigations must be delayed until this has resolved.

Barium enema classically shows the small outpouchings of diverticula and a narrowed sigmoid colon. Sigmoidoscopy can confirm inflammation, but it is poor at identifying the diverticula. A chest X-ray may show free air under the diaphragm indicating a diverticular perforation secondary to acute diverticulitis.

Management

If a patient has diverticular disease then the risk of developing diverticulitis is reduced by a high fibre diet.

Acute diverticulitis is generally treated with bed rest, IV fluids, analgesics, IV antibiotics—cefuroxime and metronidazole—and antispasmodics. Surgical intervention is only required in the minority of cases.

Possible indications for surgery include: peritonitis, fistula formation, persistent haemorrhage, pericolic abscess formation, intestinal obstruction, and repeated episodes of diverticulitis that are resistant to medical therapy.

Chronic diverticular disease is treated with a high fibre diet, antispasmodics and laxatives, e.g. ispaghula husk, nocte, lactulose 10-20 ml bd.

Diverticulitis

Diverticulitis is a condition where there is inflammation of diverticula.

Diverticulitis (acute)

Acute diverticulitis is a condition which results from acute inflammation of one or more diverticula.

This condition has a higher incidence in females than males and is most often seen in the 50-70 year old age group.

Clinical Features

Symptoms of acute diverticulitis include:

- Severe pain in the left iliac fossa or the whole of the lower abdomen which starts suddenly and is exacerbated by movement. Occasionally, the pain begins in the centre of the lower abdomen and then moves to the left.
- Slight abdominal distension.
- Nausea and anorexia.
- Constipation in most patients, a few have diarrhoea.

The patient often has along history of painful diverticular disease, flatulence, distension and left iliac fossa pain.

The general appearance is of a still patient—because of the pain—who looks flushed and feverish, with a temperature of up to 38 or 39 °C.

The abdomen moves with inspiration because the inflamed bowel is confined to its lower half.

On palpation the left iliac fossa is tender and protected by spasm of the overlying muscles. Careful palpation may detect a palpable, tender sausage-shaped mass in the left iliac fossa.

Rectal examination may cause pain as the finger is pushed high into the left side of the pelvis, especially if the inflamed colon is lying in the pelvis. The same also holds true for sigmoidoscopic examination of the recto-sigmoid junction.

Investigations

Diverticular disease is a diagnosis of exclusion. Hence, investigation must first rule out other treatable causes of similar symptomatology, e.g. ulcerative colitis, Crohn's disease, ischaemic colitis and colorectal carcinoma. Hence, barium meal, barium enema and sigmoidoscopy are common first-line investigations.

If acute inflammation is suspected, e.g. due to the presence of fever, leucocytosis and acute pain, these investigations must be delayed until this has resolved.

Barium enema classically shows the small outpouchings of diverticula and a narrowed sigmoid colon. Sigmoidoscopy can confirm inflammation, but it is poor at identifying the diverticula. A chest X-ray may show free air under the diaphragm indicating a diverticular perforation secondary to acute diverticulitis.

Management

If a patient has diverticular disease then the risk of developing diverticulitis is reduced by a high fibre diet.

Acute diverticulitis is generally treated with bed rest, IV fluids, analgesics, IV antibiotics—cefuroxime and metronidazole—and antispasmodics. Surgical intervention is only required in the minority of cases.

Possible indications for surgery include: peritonitis, fistula formation, persistent haemorrhage, pericolic abscess formation, intestinal obstruction, and repeated episodes of diverticulitis that are resistant to medical therapy.

Chronic diverticular disease is treated with a high fibre diet, antispasmodics and laxatives, e.g. ispaghula husk, nocte, lactulose 10-20 ml bd.

Diverticulitis (chronic)

Chronic diverticulits results from inflammation of one or more diverticula.

This condition exactly mimics the local clinical features of carcinoma of the colon:

- There may be diarrhoea alternating with constipation which progresses to large bowel obstruction with vomiting, distension, colicky abdominal pain and constipation—note that small bowel obstruction from adhesion of a loop of small intestine to the inflammatory mass is not uncommon.
- There may be episodes of pain in the left iliac fossa.
- Passage of mucus or bright red blood per rectum or melaena.

- Anaemia due to chronic occult bleeding. Examination reveals tenderness in the LIF and there is often a thickened mass in the region of the sigmoid colon, which may also be felt on PR.

Clinical Features

Chronic diverticulitis exactly mimics the local clinical features of carcinoma of the colon:

- There may be diarrhoea alternating with constipation which progresses to large bowel obstruction with vomiting, distension, colicky abdominal pain and constipation—note that small bowel obstruction from adhesion of a loop of small intestine to the inflammatory mass is not uncommon.
- There may be episodes of pain in the left iliac fossa, and more rarely pain elsewhere in the abdomen.
- Passage of mucus, profuse bright red blood per rectum or melaena.
- Anaemia due to chronic occult bleeding.

Examination reveals tenderness in the left iliac and there is often a thickened mass in the region of the sigmoid colon that may also be felt on rectal examination.

Investigations

Diverticular disease is a diagnosis of exclusion. Hence, investigation must first rule out other treatable causes of similar symptomatology, e.g. ulcerative colitis, Crohn's disease, ischaemic colitis and colorectal carcinoma. Hence, barium meal, barium enema and sigmoidoscopy are common first-line investigations.

If acute inflammation is suspected, e.g. due to the presence of fever, leucocytosis and acute pain, these investigations must be delayed until this has resolved.

Barium enema classically shows the small outpouchings of diverticula and a narrowed sigmoid colon. Sigmoidoscopy can confirm inflammation, but it is poor at identifying the diverticula. A chest X-ray may show free air under the diaphragm indicating a diverticular perforation secondary to acute diverticulitis.

MANAGEMENT

Chronic diverticular disease is treated with a high fibre diet, antispasmodics and laxatives, e.g. ispaghula husk, nocte, lactulose 10-20 ml bd.

Familial Polyposis Coli

Familial polyposis coli is characterized by the presence of 100 to more than 1000 tubular adenomas which carpet the colon. Less frequently, lesions occur in the stomach and the small bowel, particularly the duodenum.

This condition has a prevalence of 1 in 7000 to 1 in 24000, and is most commonly inherited in an autosomal dominant fashion, although one-third of cases are sporadic. The adenomatous polyposis gene is located on the long arm of chromosome 5.

The polyps usually appear in the second and third decade and have 100% malignant potential. Bleeding usually heralds malignant change and a poor prognosis.

Extra-gastrointestinal lesions may occur in variants.

Associated Extracolonic Tumours

Extracolonic tumours occur more often in patients with familial adenomatous polyposis than the general population. Tumours that have an increased incidence include:

- Papillary thyroid cancer
- Carcinoid tumours of the ileum
- Carcinomas of the upper gastrointestinal tract
- Medulloblastomas
- Glioblastomas.

Ocular Manifestations

Congenital hypertrophy of the retinal pigment epithelium (CHRPE) is a common fundoscopic finding in familial polyposis coli.

A recent study found the prevelance of CHPRE in patients with FAP 63.5% but only 1.2% in patients' unaffected relatives (p=0.001).

Management

Colectomy of varying degrees is necessary for familial polyposis coli as otherwise all patients develop adenocarcinoma by the age of 40 years and in about half of all cases, these malignancies are multiple. The surgical options are:

- Proctocolectomy and ileostomy:
  - abolishes the risk of large bowel cancer
  - a stoma is required, presenting psychological problems.
- Colectomy and ileorectal anastomosis:
  - does not abolish the risk of large bowel cancer
  - lifelong 6 monthly surveillance of the rectal stump is mandatory.
- Proctocolectomy and ileoanal pouch:
  - abolishes the risk of large bowel cancer
  - preferred by patients to ileostomy
  - functionally inferior, and more prone to operative complications.

The offspring of affected patients should be carefully screened on a periodic basis until about the age of 35 by colonoscopy and double contrast barium enemas. Testing for faecal occult blood is insufficient. Although polyps rarely develop before puberty, it is useful to see children with a family history before this time in order to accustomise them to the reasons for screening.

Ulcerative Colitis

Ulcerative colitis is a chronic disease of unknown aetiology in which a part or the whole of the mucosa of the large bowel becomes diffusely inflamed and may ulcerate, as a result of which the patient suffers from diarrhoea which may be bloody.

It is characterised by exacerbations and remissions.

The highest incidence of this disease is in adulthood, although it may occur in childhood.

The cause of ulcerative colitis is unknown but genetic, immunological, dietary, and psychological factors have all been implicated.

Epidemiology

This condition may occur at any time from early childhood to late adulthood.

There is an annual incidence of 5-8/100,000 in most communities of Celtic and Anglo-Saxon origin in north-western Europe, North America and New Zealand. The prevalence of symptomatic disease in north-western Europe is 70-150/100,000. This disease is very uncommon in Asia and Africa. As in Crohn's disease, familial clustering may be seen.

Pathological Features

Ulcerative colitis primarily affects the mucosa and the submucosa, with inflammatory cell infiltrate, crypt abscess and ulcer formation. Goblet cells are few in number and frequently depleted of mucus. Redundant mucosa between ulcers form pseudopolyps, and the mucosa is friable and bleeding easily on contact.

There are no skip lesions.

The rectosigmoid is most commonly involved with 50% of patients having total colonic involvement.

Chronic disease causes shortening and thickening of the bowel wall with haustral loss.

Clinical Features

Ulcerative colitis may be fulminant, chronic, or relapsing. The patient may present dehydrated and/ or toxic.

Symptoms include:

- Number of stools may vary from 1 or 2 to 20 or 30 per day.
- Diarrhoea, sometimes bloody; mild abdominal pain in the left iliac fossa; fever; weight loss.
- If this condition occurs in infancy or childhood, then the presentation may be of failure to thrive or failure to progress normally into puberty.
- In fulminating disease the presentation may be of abdominal distension, catastrophic diarrhoea, fever and collapse.

Signs may be as follows:

- Pallor, dehydration, mouth ulcers, abdominal tenderness.

Associated conditions include:

- Erythema nodosum
- Pyoderma gangrenosum
- Uveitis
- Arthritis.

Severity

The severity of ulcerative colitis can be assessed on the basis of:

- Bowel frequency—less than four motions per day is considered mild, more than six is severe.
- Rectal bleeding
- Temperature—patients with mild disease are apyrexia!, those with severe disease may be higher than 37.8 °C.
- Haemoglobin of less than 10.5 is considered severe, greater than 11 is mild.
- ESR of less than 30mm per hour is mild, greater than this is severe.
- Tachycardia is related to severity.
- Low albumin—below 30g per litre implies severe disease.

Differential Diagnosis

The differential diagnosis is influenced by the presentation, a principal factor being the age.

- Crohn's disease.
- Infective colitis is often a cause of one episode of colitis which is mislabelled as ulcerative colitis e.g. salmonellosis, shigellosis, Campylobacter, amoebiasis. In the immunosuppressed patient then one must consider opportunistic infections e.g. cytomegalovirus, herpes virus, Cryptosporidium, Mycobacterium avium intracellulare.
- Colonic carcinoma, adenoma—diagnosed on endoscopy, particularly important in the elderly.
- Diverticulitis—not in childhood.
- Irritable bowel disease, which would tend to occur in the young, and has early morning explosiveness, not tending to be bothered at night.
- Ischaemic colitis—these patients may have a history of vascular disease with sudden onset of pain, and thumb printing on plain abdominal radiography or barium enema. It does not occur in childhood.
- Post-radiation colitis, the diagnosis of which is based on the history.

Investigations

- FBC—anaemia due to blood loss; leukocytosis.
- ESR—increased; correlates with active disease.
- CRP—raised; but less so than in Crohn's disease
- biochemistry—in active disease, biochemical abnormalities may include hypokalaemia, hyponatraemia, hypomagnesaemia, hypocalcaemia, and hyoalbuminaemia. Abnormal LFTs due to associated chronic active hepatitis—increased ALT—or sclerosing cholangitis—increased alkaline phosphatase.
- ANCA—found in HLA-DR2 associated form of ulcerative colitis.

- Radiology:
  - plain abdominal x-ray—excludes toxic dilatation, which is more than 5.5 cm in diameter in adults
  - barium enema:
    - § diagnosis of extent and severity of the disease
    - § procedure is contraindicated in those patients at risk of a toxic dilatation.
- Rectal biopsy—taken at sigmoidoscopy.
- Colonoscopy—this is contraindicated in those patients at risk of toxic dilatation. Allows multiple biopsies to be taken throughout the colon and delineation of the extent and activity of the disease.
- White cell scan—allows imaging in severe disease.
- Molecular biology—a high intensity of CD44v6 and v3 epitope expression on crypt epithelial cells in patients with UC has been noted. This observation may have diagnostic potential in distinguishing UC from Crohn's.

Diagnosis of Ulcerative Colitis

Careful history and examination is, of course, very important for the diagnosis of ulcerative colitis. The hallmark is bloody diarrhoea with mucus, usually of gradual onset, but it can be abrupt.

The diagnosis of ulcerative colitis is based on:

- Exclusion of other causes of diarrhoea like bacillary or amoebic dysentry.
- Colonoscopy and biopsy—histological characteristics, and endoscopic features.
- Differentiation from Crohn's disease—this may be very difficult:
  - ANCA positivity associated with forms of ulcerative colitis.
  - increased expression of CD44v6 and CD44v3 variants in the colonic mucosa of patients with ulcerative colitis has been described and may have diagnostic potential in differentiating

ulcerative colitis and Crohn's disease. There is absence of CD44v6 expression from normal colonic mucosa, but CD44v6 and CD44v3 have been identified in colorectal tumours.

Management

There have been massive improvements in the management of ulcerative colitis in the past 40 or 50 years, as evidenced by the death rates in severe attacks:

- Before 1952, 45%
- Now, 1 to 2 %.

The management has been improved by:

- Corticosteroids.
- Better understanding of fluid balance and electrolytes in severely ill patients.
- Better understanding of indicators of severity of the disease.

Note that all the management strategies listed here require considerable modification in children.

Local complications of ulcerative colitis include:

- Haemorrhage
- Malnutrition
- Electrolyte imbalance
- Toxic megacolon
- Stricture formation—rare
- Fistula formation—rare
- Perforation
- Increased risk of malignancy—lymphoma, carcinoma.

General complications include:

- Weight loss
- Anaemia
- Hypoproteinaemia
- Arthropathy—tends to affect large weight-bearing joints

- Liver associations:
  - primary sclerosing cholangitis
  - fatty liver
  - non-specific hepatitis
  - pericholangitis
  - chronic active hepatitis
  - bile duct carcinoma.
- Sacro-iliitis and ankylosing spondylitis.
- Pyoderma gangrenosum.
- Erythema nodosum.
- Anterior uveitis.
- Episcleritis.
- Carcinoma of the bile ducts—rare.

Note that **gallstones are associated with Crohn's disease but not ulcerative colitis.**

Prognosis

The prognosis of ulcerative colitis:

- A colectomy is curative.
- Seventy percent of patients with untreated UC relapse annually.
- There is a 1% risk of the development of colonic cancer if someone has the disease for 10 years; in most UK centres, patients with extensive UC of 10 years' duration are offered colonoscopy every 1-2 years in an effort to prevent colonic cancer by taking multiple biopsies to look for mucosal dysplasia and to offer colectomy if appropriate, or to detect cancer at a curable stage (1).
- There is a substantial variation in severity, extent and responsiveness, together with extra-intestinal and multiple intestinal manifestations.
- Life-expectancy is similar to that of the general population.
- Patients with well-controlled distal UC can be followed up routinely in primary care (will require a blood count and liver function test every 6-12 months, and referral for colonoscopy at 8-10 years to reassess disease extent).

Ischaemic Colitis

Ischaemic colitis is typically, a chronic segmental process in elderly patients affecting the watershed areas of the splenic flexure or rectosigmoid area. It is caused by transient critical ischaemia.

The condition may resolve. In others, stricture develops which requires surgical resection.

Aetiology

The most common cause is arterial occlusion, usually of the superior mesenteric artery.

Classification:

- Thromboembolic arterial occlusion.
- Mesenteric venous occlusion.
- Systemic vasculitis.
- Cardiovascular causes.
- Secondary to intestinal obstruction
  - strangulated hernia
  - intussusception—usually in children
  - volvulus—usually small bowel or sigmoid colon.

Clinical Features

There is often a history of vascular disease or diabetes, and it sometimes may follow aneurysm surgery and ligation of the inferior mesenteric artery.

Patients usually complain of cramp-like, left sided abdominal pain which lasts for a few hours, and is followed by rectal bleeding. The bleeding is dark red, often without faeces, and may occur 2-3 times over a period of 12 hours.

There are **no abdominal masses.**

It may be difficult to distinguish the bleeding of ischaemic colitis from that due to inflammatory bowel disease, diverticulitis or carcinoma.

Diagnosis is usually established on the basis of:

- Plain abdominal x-ray—may reveal mucosal oedema at the splenic flexure, so called "thumb printing"; a single segment is affected with symmetrical stricture.

- Barium enema—support x-ray findings; contra-indicated in acute illness because of risk of perforation.
- Endoscopy—variable appearance from mild reddening to gangrene.
- Histology:
  - intramucosal haemorrhage
  - fibrosis
  - haemosiderin—uncommon.

Mesenteric Adenitis

Mesenteric adenitis is an important cause of right iliac fossa pain in children, and as such is important as a differential diagnosis of appendicitis. It is due to non-specific inflammation of the mesenteric lymph nodes which provokes a mild peritoneal reaction and stimulates painful peristalsis in the terminal ileum.

Clinical Features

The individual with mesenteric adenitis is usually under 30 years of age and presents with abdominal pain, which may be generalised or localised, possibly in the right iliac fossa. There is little guarding or rebound, and moderate tenderness. The patient may be pyrexial and there may be diarrhoea, with or without vomiting, or a recent upper respiratory tract infection.

Differential Diagnosis

The important differential for mesenteric adenitis is acute appendicitis, but the clinical picture of this condition can usually be discriminated from the absence of rectal tenderness, and a temperature higher than 38.5 degees C. However, if there is uncertainty, a laparotomy may be performed. Adenitis is confirmed by a normal appendix and large inflamed, fleshy lymph nodes in the mesentery.

Volvulus

A volvulus is the twisting of a loop of bowel around its mesenteric axis. This process results in a combination of obstruction together with occlusion of the main vessels at the base of the involved mesentery.

This condition most commonly affects the sigmoid, caecum and the small intestine. Rare forms of volvulus affect the gallbladder and the stomach.

If the condition is not corrected, the obstructed bowel becomes necrotic, peritonitis and rupture of the bowel occur, and death may ensue.

RECTAL DISEASES AND CONDITIONS

Rectal Carcinoma

Rectal carcinoma affects both sexes equally. It is most common in the 50-70 year old age group; however, any age from about the twenties upwards may be affected.

Rectal carcinoma accounts for about a third of tumours of the large intestine.

Possible predisposing factors include ulcerative colitis, familial polyposis and pre-existing adenoma.

The vast majority of carcinomas are adenocarcinomas.

Macroscopically, rectal carcinomas are usually ulcerating. Stenosing rectal carcinomas may occur at the recto-sigmoid junction. Rectal carcinomas may also be colloidal or papilliferous.

Clinical Features

The clinical features of rectal carcinoma include:

- Rectal bleeding:
  - haematochezia—passage of bright red blood with bowel movements
  - the bleeding is commonly persistent but rarely copious
  - may be streaked on stool or mixed with mucous.

- Change in bowel habit; low tumours cause slight constipation but high tumours cause alternating constipation and diarrhoea.
- Tenesmus.
- Generalised debility and malaise.

Less common features include:

- Pain:
  - colic, with distension and vomiting, due to lumen obstruction, or
  - pain localised to rectum, due to direct spread to surrounding structures, especially the sacral nerves,
  - rarely, pain during defaecation
- Ascites
- Abdominal distension
- Hepatomegaly.

In 90% of cases, rectal examination reveals the carcinoma:

- Papilliferous tumours feel soft, frond like, and have a narrow pedicle
- Villous carcinomata are often impalpable
- Carcinomatous ulcers feel hard and bulge into the lumen of the rectum. Their base is irregular and friable, and they usually have an everted edge.

Tumour Suppressor Genes and Colorectal Carcinoma

Several tumour suppressor genes have been identified as being involved in tumour initiation and progression:

- Inactivation of the DCC gene:
  - DCC stands for Deleted in Colon Cancer
  - on chromosome 18q
  - DCC is a membrane-bound protein that shares sequence homology with neural adhesion molecules (N-CAM)
  - DCC is xpressed in the axons of peripheral and central neurons and in differentiated cells of the intestine

- DCC mutations have only been found in sporadic colorectal cancers.
- APC:
  - the Adenomatous Polyposis Colon gene
  - mutations of the APC tumour suppressor gene are unique to colorectal carcinomas.
- MutHLS homology genes:
  - these proteins are involved in mismatch repair of DNA
  - dysfunction results in the hereditary non-polyposis colorectal cancer.

Treatment of Rectal Carcinoma

The treatment of rectal cancer is usually by surgery.

Radiotherapy and cytotoxic chemotherapy are used palliatively where the tumour is inoperable.

Colorectal carcinomas are relatively unresponsive to chemotherapy but palliative chemotherapy in patients with locally advanced or metastatic disease has been shown to reduce death and progression at 12 months . The findings translate into a 16% absolute difference in survival and a 25% increase in progression free survival (increases in 3.7 months in median survival and 6 months in median progression free survival) in patients treated with palliative chemotherapy e.g. 5-fluorouracil alone or in combination with other chemotherapeutic agents.

Surgical treatments

The choice of operation depends on the height of the lesion above the anal verge, it's configuration, gross extent and degree of differentiation, and the patient's general condition. A colostomy may be required and this should be discussed with the patient.

Four principal operations are used:

- **Local resection**: if the patient is too old or frail to withstand a major operation

- **Anterior resection of rectum**: for growths more than 10 cm from the anal verge but below the recto-sigmoid junction.
- **Abdomino-perineal resection of rectum**: for growths less than 10 cm from the anal verge.
- **Hartmann's procedure**: if the tumour is unresectable.

Haemorrhoids

Anal continence requires the apposition of three mucosal pads which:
- Are composed of subepithelial vascular cushions.
- Are found in the left lateral, right anterolateral and right posterolateral portions of the anal canal.
- Form haemorrhoids when the pads become enlarged and congested.

Haemorrhoids may cause:
- Anal pain
- Pruritus ani
- Bright red rectal bleeding

Haemorrhoids are very common and can occur at any age.

Aetiology

The causes of haemorrhoids is not well understood but the following factors are important:
- Constipation and prolonged straining at stool
  - the typical Western diet is low in fibre and haemorrhoids are more common.
  - haemorrhoids are uncommon in developing countries.
- Increased anal sphincter tone:
  - several effective treatments aim to reduce anal tone, including anal stretch procedures and nitroglycerine ointment.
- Obstruction of venous flow may play a role:
  - during pregnancy
  - in patients with portal hypertension.

Classification of Haemorrhoids

Haemorrhoids may be either:

- Internal:
  - with an origin above the dentate line
  - are generally painless
- External:
  - with an origin below the dentate line
  - are generally painfull.

Haemorrhoids may be of four grades:

- Grade I:
  - do not prolapse out of the anal canal
- Grade II:
  - prolapse on defecation but reduce spontaneously
- Grade III:
  - require manual reduction
- Grade IV:
  - cannot be reduced.

Clinical Features

Haemorrhoids often only produce intermittent symptoms. Symptomatic episodes are often precipitated by constipation. These episodes usually last from a few days to a few weeks. Often they are completely asymptomatic between episodes.

Clinical Features of piles include:

- Bleeding after defaecation:
  - may just stain the toilet paper or streak the faeces,
  - if copious it may splash around the lavatory pan.
- Faecal soiling.
- Mucus discharge.
- Pruritus ani.
- Occasionally pain:
  - thrombosis may cause acute severe anal pain occasionally necessitating hospital admission.
- Grades 2-4 may be felt as a rectal mass.

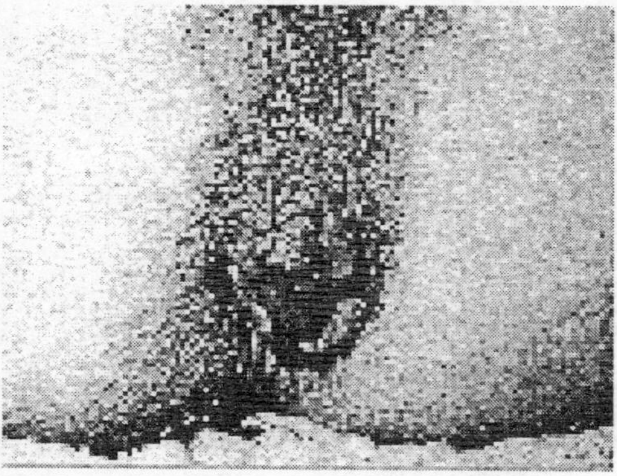

Fig. 8.1: Third degree haemorrhoids

Differential Diagnosis

The other common cause of a localised anal swelling is the perianal haematoma. This lesion is always covered by skin, which distinguishes it from the mucosa-covered prolapsed haemorrhoid.

Another cause of bright red blood passed per rectum associated with the passing of stools is an anal fissure.

Other differentials are:

- Rectal prolapse
- Anal polyp
- Inflammatory bowel disease
- Rectal carcinoma.

Investigations

Suspected haemorrhoids are investigated by:

- Examine the abdomen, groins and genitals for masses, lymphadenopathy, etc.
- Digital examination:
  - this is essential
  - helps to exclude carcinoma and provides a useful measure of anal tone
  - note that haemorrhoids are often not palpable on digital examination because they empty with pressure from the examining finger.

- Proctoscopy:
  - necessary to diagnose first or second degree piles
  - piles are seen bulging into the lumen as the proctoscope is withdrawn.
- Sigmoidoscopy:
  - indicated if there is a history of bleeding or there are symptoms that are suspicious of malignancy.

Strangulated Haemorrhoids

Infarcted haemorrhoids are the result of infarction within the venous saccules of the anal cushions. They are sometimes termed 'strangulated' even though the cushions become engorged as opposed to devoid of blood.

The patient reports severe pain and discomfort at the site. There may be local swelling. The haemorrhoid appears black-blue and there may be local oedema.

The treatment of choice is bed rest, analgesia and stool softeners to limit straining. Reduction of the haemorrhoid has little effect on pain. Most infarcted haemorrhoids do not require surgical intervention but instead the symptoms resolve with time. If there is frank and widespread necrosis, local debridement may be undertaken to reduce discomfort.

Management

The best management is prevention.

The active treatment of haemorrhoids includes:

- Conservative treatment
- Surgical treatment.

Conservative Treatment

Other measures include:

- Ensuring the perineum is dried and washed after defaecation:
  - these measures help to prevent/treat pruritus ani

  - the application of talcum powder after cleaning is a simple measure that will keep the perineum dry
- Digital replacement of prolapsed haemorrhoids:
  - this can lead to symptomatic relief.
- Local anaesthetic creams and ointments
- Treatment aimed at reducing spasm of the internal anal sphincter:
  - nitroglycerine ointments:
    - § glyceryl trinitrate 0.2-0.3% (unlicensed)
  - botulinum toxin injection

The *surgical treatment* may be divided into:

Outpatient Interventions for Haemorrhoids

Outpatient interventions for treating haemorrhoids include:

- Sclerotherapy
- Rubber band ligation
- Photocoagulation
- Cryotherapy.

These treatments are appropriate for:

- Patients with small haemorrhoids (grade I or II)
- Patients with larger piles who do not wish to undergo inpatient treatment

The treatment must be applied as high as possible avoid excessive discomfort. There may be some minor bleeding following treatment.

Inpatient Interventions for Haemorrhoids

Inpatient interventions for haemorrhoids include:

- Gentle anal dilatation under general anaesthetic:
  - Lord's stretch procedure
- Haemorrhoidectomy.

Rectal Prolapse

Rectal prolapse is a condition that occurs in two main groups, young children and the elderly. In children, it is generally a relatively minor and self-correcting problem, but there are some important aetiologies to exclude.

The rest of this section of the system will discuss rectal prolapse in adults.

Pathogenesis

A rectal prolapse is in effect a hernia of the rectum through the floor of the pelvis. The mucosa and muscle wall of the rectum intussuscept through the anal canal. Contributory factors include denervation of the puborectalis muscle, loss of the acute anorectal angle, and poor fixation of the rectum to the sacrum. Early on in the condition, prolapse only occurs with defaecation and retracts spontaneously. As the condition worsens, rectal prolapse may occur with only slight increases in intra-abdominal pressure, e.g. when the patient stands up.

Aetiology

There are a couple of important aetiologies to consider in children:

- Cystic fibrosis
- Chronic malabsorptive states, including coeliac disease.

Clinical Features

The patient with a rectal prolapse is usually elderly and female. The peak age for onset in males is between 20-40 years of age.

The patient complains of a variable length of 'something' coming down their back passage when they defaecate. It causes a profuse discharge of mucous which soils the patients underclothes. There may also be rectal bleeding.

As the condition becomes more advanced then the prolapse may come down more readily. The patient may find it impossible to get outside the house and may become socially isolated.

On examination, the prolapse will appear when the patient strains; this is best achieved with the patient sitting forward on a toilet to cover the eventuality of incontinence. High in the rectum at sigmoidoscopy, toilet paper may be sighted. This is a very accurate indicator of prolapse as the paper was used to replace the apex of the prolapse.

Note, rectal prolapse may also result as a complication of injury during a forceps delivery.

Investigations

The following series of investigations may be of value for rectal prolapse:

- Sigmoidoscopy:
  - this may show lavatory paper in the rectum that has been used to replace the prolapse
  - traumatic proctitis may be revealed.
- Proctoscopy:
  - the prolapse will be seen to fill the lumen
- Anorectal manometry:
  - intraluminal pressures in the anus and rectum can be measured at different levels with the sphincters lax and also maximally contracted
  - the results are compared to normal controls.
- Evacuation proctography:
  - demonstrates an increased anorectal angle, occlusion of the rectal canal or recto-recto intussusception.

Management

The elderly patient will either conceal a rectal prolapse, or tolerate it remarkably. Some patients become accustomed to pushing back the prolapse after defaecation and rarely complain about their condition.

Conservative management is of little benefit. A high fibre diet is of little help because the problem has progressed to an anatomical defect that will never spontaneously recover. Other forms of conservative management include stool softeners and perineal exercises.

Surgical Management

- The usual operation for a rectal prolapse is designed to secure the rectum in the abdominal cavity or pelvis. The two most commonly used procedures have an abdominal approach: the **Wells operation** and the **Ripstein rectoplexy.**

If an abdominal operation is contraindicated then a subcutaneous circum-anal silicone rubber ring may be inserted. However, this may cause problems if it is too loose—recurrent prolapse—or too tight—causing constipation.

Delorme's operation is a successful alternative in the **elderly** individual.

ANAL AND PERIANAL DISEASES AND CONDITIONS

Anal Fistula

An anal fistula is an abnormal communication between the perianal skin and the anal or rectal lumen. It may occur as a complication of an anal abscess that has burst on to the skin, or may occur after incomplete surgical drainage.

Fistulae are described according to the level at which they transgress the anal sphincters. If the internal orifice of the fistula begins below puborectalis, then this is known as a 'low' fistula. If the internal orifice begins above puborectalis then the fistula is described as 'high'. High anal fistulas are much rarer than low fistulas, occurring in Crohn's disease, ulcerative colitis—more rarely, or as a result of a foreign body. The management of a high fistula is more complex than that of a low fistula.

Clinical Features

The patient with a perianal fistula complains of intermittent discharge in the perianal region, perianal discomfort, and chronic irritation.

On examination, the external opening of the fissure is generally seen lateral to the anus. The external opening may be seen as a small papilla of granulation tissue. Note that though this clinical picture is diagnostic of an anal fistula, often the apparently trivial skin lesion may be diagnosed as a pustule. The internal opening to the fistula may be felt on rectal examination.

Examination with a proctoscope may allow direct visualisation of the internal opening. It may be possible to pass a probe along the course of the fistula to chart its pathway.

Goodsall's Rule

Goodsall's rule is applied to the examination of anal fistula. It states that if the fistula lies in the anterior half of the anal area then it opens directly into the anal canal, while if a fistula lies in the posterior half of the canal then it tracks around the anus laterally and opens into the midline posteriorly.

Management

The form of management of an anal fistula depends on whether it is a 'high' fistula, i.e. the internal opening is above puborectalis, or a 'low' fistula, where the internal opening is below this point. Management of a high fistula is more difficult because anal continence is maintained by the deep ring of the external anal sphincter and the puborectalis sling and this mechanism is at risk when a high fistula is operated on.

Low fistula: the operation involves laying open the fistula. A probe is carefully inserted into the external opening and passed into the anal canal via the internal opening. The tract is then completely laid open by cutting down on the probe. If there are any lateral extensions then these must also be laid open. The patient will be in hospital for 3-10 days and will be off work for 2-4 weeks.

High fistula: operative management of a high fistula is more complex and highly specialised. The patient will again be in hospital for 3-10 days but will be off work for a longer period 4-6 weeks.

It is possible to use a seton—a ligature of silk or linen—to lay open an intersphincteric tract. The seton acts as an irritant, and, with gradual removal, the course of the fistula fibroses. There is a high failure rate with this technique.

Complicated high fistulae may warrant the fashioning of a defunctioning proximal colostomy. If possible, Crohn's disease fistulae are treated conservatively.

Anal Fissure

An anal fissure is a crack in the wall of the anal mucosa so that the circular muscle layer is exposed. The tear usually occurs directly posteriorly and in the midline.

Men and women are equally affected. The peak incidence is in the 20-30 year old age group.

An anal fissure may be produced secondary to inflammatory bowel disease, especially Crohn's, in which case it should heal with successful medical treatment of the primary condition.

Aetiology

The most common cause of an anal fissure is the passage of a large stool after a period of constipation.

Other causes include:

- Secondary to Crohn's disease
- As a result of abuse in children

Clinical Features

The salient features of fissure in ano are:

- History of pain of defaecation—often first occurs during a period of constipation
- The passing of stools may cause sphincter spasm and acute pain during defaecation, which may persist for up to an hour

- Patient may develop a fear of defaecation which in turn aggravates the constipation; even sitting may be avoided
- There is often fresh rectal bleeding at defaecation; the patient complains of 'bright red blood on the paper'.

On examination:

- There is a longitudinal tear that nearly always occurs directly posteriorly and in the midline.
- A sentinel pile may be seen if the anus is inspected with the buttocks gently parted; the sentinel pile is the torn, bunched-up strip of mucosa at the base of the fissure.

The severity of the pain and muscle spasm may preclude digital examination and necessitate examination under general anaesthesia.

Management

Conservative management:

- Introduction of more bran into the diet together with laxatives and analgesic suppositories.
- Some suggest the use of a plastic anal dilator.
- Topical glyceryl trinitrate may be beneficial.
- Botulinum toxin injections may be used as an alternative to treatment with GTN (or in patients in whom GTN fails).
- Conservative management is inappropriate if a sentinel tag or fibroepithelial polyp is present.

Surgical management—this can bring immediate relief:

- Internal sphincterotomy:
  - in studies with short term follow-up the healing rate was 92-100%.
- Manual dilatation:
  - reduces sphincter pressure
  - results in healing in 40-70%
  - results in incontinence in 25-75%
  - is rarely indicated.

Perianal Abscess

Perianal abscesses are common surgical emergencies. They may present acutely or insidiously with perianal pain, tenderness and swelling.

Ischiorectal lesions are the commonest, but abscesses may be perianal, intermuscular or pelvirectal.

Men are affected more often than women.

Aetiology

Commonly a perianal abscess is formed as result of infection arising in a perianal gland. There are 10 to 15 of these glands lying between the internal and external anal sphincters. They drain into tiny pits at the bases of the anal columns along the dentate line. The ducts through which the glands drain are very tiny and these may become obstructed by faeces and so initiate infection. The abscess that results lies between the anal sphincters and tends to point towards the skin at the anal margin. Lateral spread may occur into the ischiorectal fossa, or rarely, superiorly above the levator ani into the pararectal fossa.

There are a variety of conditions that predispose to perianal abscesses including tuberculosis, actinomycosis, mucinous carcinoma, and inflammatory bowel disease, especially Crohn's disease.

Clinical Features

A perianal abscess may affect patients of any age.

The patient complains of a gradual onset of pain around the anus. The pain becomes more severe and throbs. The condition makes defaecation and sitting painful.

The patient may be sitting with one buttock raised, which is pathognomonic of the condition. On examination, the abscess may be seen deep in the skin next to the anus. There is localised tenderness and swelling. Proctoscopic examination may reveal the damaged opening to the affected gland—pus may be seen discharging from it.

Management

Diligent sigmoidoscopy is necessary to find the perianal abscess outlet. Pus should be sent for culture of both routine gut and skin organisms, and additionally, acid fast bacilli. Specimens of the abscess should be sent for histopathological examination.

If the abscess is caught early then treatment with oral antibiotics may abort the infection. If the abscess has become established then it requires drainage and curettage. This is performed under general anaesthesia. The patient may stay in hospital for 3-7 days and be off work for 1-4 weeks.

Pruritus Ani

Pruritus ani is itching around the anus.

Possible causes include:

- Threadworm infection—itching occurs at night and may contribute to the autoinfection of patients with this condition, especially younger patients
- Simple irritancy e.g. faecal soiling, poor hygiene
- Local disorders e.g. haemorrhoids, infection, warts; rarely, neoplasm
- Primary dermatoses e.g. psoriasis, lichen sclerosis, erythrasma
- Diabetes mellitus—predisposing to candidiasis
- Allergy to local anaesthetic
- Use of topical steroids
- Foreign bodies

Treatment in General practice

This is depends on cause.

If threadworm is suspected then treatment with mebendazole.

If clinical examination in an adult reveals excoriation and nil else then treat with a combined steroid/antibiotic/antifungal preparation (e.g. Tri-adcortyl cream) and review.

Chapter 9

Vascular Diseases and Conditions

Surgically treatable vascular diseases and conditions can be subdivided in to those which affect the arterial and those which affect the venous system.

ARTERIAL DISEASE

- Acute ischaemia
- Occlusive
- Aneurysmal
- Aortic dissection.

Acute Ischaemic Disease

Acute ischaemia describes ischaemia which is of rapid onset, and as such both stroke and myocardial infarction might be considered to belong here. This section will however deal with acute ischaemia of the following areas which are more immediately amenable to surgical treatment:

- The lower limb
- The gut
- The renal artery.

Acute Lower Limb Ischaemia

Ischaemia in the lower limb may develop acutely as a result of embolism, thrombosis or arterial occlusion by trauma or tourniquets.

Emboli frequently impact at branching points such as the aortic bifurcation—causing a saddle embolus which affects both limbs, the common femoral bifurcation, and the popliteal trifurcation.

Thrombotic occlusion may develop anywhere especially if there is pre-existing atherosclerosis. The consequences are particularly severe if it occurs in the popliteal artery where there are few useful collaterals, the external iliac or common femoral arterial trunk, which is the axial blood supply of the lower limb, or the profunda femoris.

Early diagnosis is vital since infarction can develop within hours unless treatment is instigated.

Aetiology

Acute ischaemia results principally from embolism or thrombotic occlusion in an essential distributing artery:

- Embolism—most large emboli originate in the heart, as a result of atrial fibrillation, mitral stenosis—left atrial thrombus, atrial myxoma or myocardial infarction—mural thrombus.
- Thrombotic occlusion of an artery already narrowed by atherosclerosis.
- Thrombosis of a popliteal artery aneurysm.

Rarely, acute ischaemia may result from widespread thrombosis due to:

- High oestrogen contraceptive pill
- Polycythaemia rubra vera
- Thrombocythaemia
- Leukaemia.

Clinical Features

These are the six P's:

- Pain—sudden onset, continuous, variable intensity; often at the junction of perfused and ischaemic tissue, usually in one periphery.
- Paraesthesia—sudden onset, usually in one periphery; may be an altered or a complete absence of sensation.
- Pallor—periphery is white and may become blue with onset of necrosis. There is poor peripheral

capillary return on pressure blanching and the skin may blister. Buerger's test is positive.

- Perishing cold.
- Pulselessness—foot pulses are absent, and may be undetectable by Doppler ultrasound. Popliteal and femoral pulses may be absent depending on the level of occlusion.
- Paralysis—indicates extreme ischaemia. The movements of flexion and extension of the ankle and toes are eventually lost.

Involvement of both limbs implies occlusion at the aortic bifurcation.

Clinically, it is often difficult to identify the cause of the ischaemia. An embolus is more likely if the other limb has good peripheral pulses and a normal ankle systolic pressure, or if there is a history of risk factors such as a previous myocardial infarction. Thrombosis is more likely if there is a history of claudication.

Management

This depends upon the underlying cause of the ischaemia. If an embolus is responsible an embolectomy may be performed whereas emergency reconstructive surgery, usually a femoro-popliteal or a femoro-tibial bypass, is indicated in thrombotic occlusion.

Distinguishing the two aetiologic agents is difficult, and requires a careful history and examination. Blood should be tested for predisposing blood disorders, and sent for crossmatch.

Suitable anti-coagulation therapy should be started using intravenous heparin. If an arterial embolism is suspected, this anticoagulant therapy should be continued later with oral warfarin.

Arteriography will indicate the site and nature of the obstruction, but it may take up valuable time, and in some centres is only used if there is diagnostic doubt.

Fibrinolytic agents should be considered if surgery is necessary but the patient is surgically unfit. Streptokinase may be instilled directly into a clot via an arterial catheter but should not be given systemically. Thrombolysis takes time and the clot normally dissolves within 12 to 72 hours.

Peripheral Embolic Disease of the Gut

Acute ischaemia of the gut is characterised by:
- Severe abdominal pain
- Vomiting
- Possibly, passage of blood per rectum
- Sign of peritonitis and obstruction
  The patient deteriorates rapidly.
  Diagnosis is confirmed at laparotomy.

Treatment

The embolus should be removed if possible.

This involves embolectomy and revascularisation of the gut immediately. If this is impossible or unsuccessful then the infarcted gut must be removed surgically.

Secondary prevention includes:
- Anticoagulation
- Control of any condition such as atrial fibrillation
- Aspirin therapy—75 mg per day.

Peripheral Embolic Disease of the Kidney

The severe loin pain and haematuria of a renal embolus may mimic a renal stone.

An IVP should distinguish between the two diagnoses.

Selective renal arteriography will confirm the arterial occlusion.

Treatment

Treatment is surgical. Depending on the viability of the affected kidney, an embolectomy or a nephrectomy is performed.

Secondary prevention management options include:

- Anticoagulation
- Control of any condition such as atrial fibrillation
- Aspirin therapy—75 mg per day.

Occlusive Vascular Disease

Occlusive vascular disease is most commonly due to atherosclerosis and it affects arteries leading to distal arterial insufficiency and ischaemia.

Peripheral Arterial Disease(PAD)

Peripheral Arterial Disease (PAD) includes disorders that obstruct arterial blood flow, excluding the coronary and intracranial circulations.

Peripheral Arterial Disease affecting the legs is of overwhelming importance and is the focus of this section.

There are several stages in the severity of PAD in the lower limb:

- Intermittent claudication:
  - pain, usually in the calf, that is precipitated by walking
- Rest pain:
  - pain, usually in the foot, that is worse elevated in bed at night and is relieved by lowering the leg
- Arterial ulceration of the leg and foot
- Gangrene of the leg and foot.

Rest pain, ulceration or gangrene indicates critical limb ischaemia. Critical limb ischaemia has a high risk of amputation and death.

Aetiology

The most common cause is atherosclerosis.

Other rarer causes of large vessel arterial disease include:

- giant cell arteritis
- Buerger's disease
- Takayasu's disease.

Buerger's Disease

Buerger's disease typically occurs in heavy smokers who started smoking at an early age. It begins in young adult life, usually between 20 and 35 years of age, and historically, has been regarded as a male disease. However, several cases have now been reported both in women, perhaps coincidental with the increase in women smokers, and in non-smokers.

Pathology

In the acute stage, thrombosis occurs in small and medium sized arteries and veins. Unlike arteriosclerosis, digital vessels are commonly involved. Dense aggregates of polymononuclear leukocytes are seen within the thrombus. There is no necrosis of the arterial wall unlike in arteriosclerosis or polyarteritis nodosa. Later, microabscesses are observed and giant cells appear within the granulation tissue. The thrombus is organised and its lumen may be re-canalised.

Older lesions show chronic inflammatory infiltrates or extensive fibrosis. Peripheral nerves may be involved in addition to arteries and veins.

Aetiology

There is a striking association with smoking but a causal relationship has yet to be demonstrated. Current belief is that the disease is caused by an immunologic process initiated in response to smoking and other factors.

Socio-economic group may be important since many patients come from poor backgrounds with inadequate hygiene and a history of chronic fungal infection. Genetic factors are suggested by the fact that blacks are rarely affected whereas the disease is common in Asia. Autonomic overactivity is suggested by the association with severe peripheral vasospasm and hyperhidrosis. Familial predisposition has also been reported.

Clinical Features

The clinical course of the disease is often protracted and extremely painful but usually remits if the patient stops smoking.

Major features may include:

- Peripheral ischaemia:
  - especially of the upper extremities
  - ischaemic areas are sharply demarcated from adjacent, well-perfused tissue
- Faint/absent pulses in small and medium sized arteries-commonly, radials, tibials and plantars; rarely, brachials or femorals
- Foot claudication
- Superficial thrombophlebitis
- Cold sensitivity
- Raynaud's phenomenon
- Peripheral neuropathy
- Gangrene of the toes and fingers.

Investigations

A formal vascular assessment should be undertaken e.g. ESR, fibrinogen levels, platelets, etc. Serological tests may be undertaken to exclude autoimmune diseases.

Arteriography reveals segmental obliteration of arteries, especially the medium sized arteries of the forearm and calf, with a strikingly normal appearance of the remaining vessels. Digital arteries are frequently involved. The femoral arteries may show a characteristic "corrugation".

Digital plethysmography may reveal small vessel occlusions.

Differential Diagnosis

This includes:

- Arteriosclerosis—but unlikely to cause small vessel disease and characterised by irregular atherosclerotic plaques
- systemic lupus erythematous

Treatment

The patient should be advised to give up smoking since indefinite remissions often follow abstinence from cigarettes. Reduction in smoking is not sufficient.

Pain control is a major problem. Narcotics are usually necessary despite the risk of addiction. Peripheral or sympathetic nerve blocks may provide temporary relief. Cervical or lumbar sympathectomy may be of benefit. Severe, persistent pain may warrant amputation even in the absence of tissue necrosis.

Arterial reconstruction is usually impossible because of the distal nature of the disease. Reconstructions for Buerger's disease also have a higher failure rate than comparable reconstructions for arteriosclerosis.

Management Of PAD

Management is dependent on the severity of the symptoms and the extent to which they affect the patient's life. Options range from little or no active intervention in mild claudication to amputation in critical ischaemia.

Mild to Moderate Claudication

Management is generally conservative, as in one-third of patients, symptoms resolve spontaneously.

Measures are aimed at preventing disease progression:

- Exclude any treatable underlying disease e.g. diabetes mellitus
- Encourage the patient to stop smoking and /or lose weight as appropriate and/or manage hyperlipidaemia
- Encourage regular exercise to open and develop the collateral circulation. Exercise tolerance may be improved by using a walking stick and walking more slowly.

- Emphasize the need to take great care not to injure the leg since healing is generally poor.
- Investigate and treat any systemic manifestations of atherosclerosis.
- Drug therapy—anti-platelet drugs such as aspirin, may, long-term, improve outcome
- follow-up patients regularly.

Disabling Claudication

Patients with disabling claudication have either:

- Worsening claudication e.g. decreased exercise tolerance.
- Claudication that interferes with everyday life.

The preferred treatment depends upon the severity of the disease and the overall fitness of the patient. Options include:

- Percutaneous balloon angioplasty
- Local fibrinolytic therapy e.g. streptokinase 6000 units per hour, delivered directly through a catheter
- Reconstructive arterial surgery.

Critical Ischaemia

Patients with severe ischaemia have symptoms such as rest pain or skin necrosis. The extent of the arterial insufficiency can be assessed by doppler pressure index studies and arteriography.

Treatment options include:

- IV drug therapy e.g. vasodilators
- Lumbar sympathectomy
- Percutaneous balloon angioplasty
- Reconstructive arterial surgery
- Amputation
- Terminal pain relief.

Mesenteric Ischaemia

Ischaemic bowel disease may be acute or chronic. Most cases result from arterial occlusion, usually of the superior mesenteric artery.

The small bowel is affected uncommonly. Ischaemic injury to the large bowel may be referred to as ischaemic colitis.

Anatomy and Physiology

Relevant blood supply:

- Coeliac axis—first portion of the duodenum
- Superior mesenteric artery—the remainder of the small bowel and the large bowel up to the splenic flexure
- Inferior mesenteric artery—the remainder of the large bowel and part of the rectum
- Branches of the internal iliac artery—distal rectum.

Potential areas of ischaemia:

- Splenic flexure—watershed between the superior and inferior mesenteric arteries
- Rectosigmoid region—watershed between the inferior mesenteric artery and the branches from the internal iliac artery.

Normally, the intra-abdominal digestive organs receive 25% of the cardiac output. Hypotension causes mesenteric arterial occlusion with shunting of the blood to the heart and brain. The bowel can tolerate a 70% reduction in blood supply without damage. The mucosa is the most vulnerable area; the muscularis propria, the least.

Ischaemia, i.e. an inadequate blood supply, results in tissue hypoxia and the accumulation of toxic waste products, which may cause tissue necrosis, i.e. infarction.

The degree of bowel damage sustained depends upon:

- Rapidity of the ischaemia and its duration
- Extent of any collaterals
- Metabolic requirements of the area affected
- Nature of bowel flora—for example, anaerobes such as Clostridia species may produce toxins that accentuate damage.

Pathology

The pathological features depend on the severity of the ischaemia.

The affected bowel appears red or purple. It is often moist and dilated with a friable often haemorrhagic mucosa. The wall may tear easily and perforate.

In less severe lesions, there is mucosal necrosis which is reversible. The mucosa will regenerate if the blood supply can be restored.

In more severe injury, the muscularis propria is damaged. Any healing results in stricture.

Classification

- Acute mesenteric ischaemia—predominantly, the superior mesenteric artery
- Chronic mesenteric ischaemia
- Ischaemic colitis.

Superior Mesenteric Artery Occlusion

The superior mesenteric artery is the gastrointestinal artery most commonly involved in acute, occlusive events leading to ischaemia. It supplies the small bowel apart from the proximal duodenum and drains via the superior mesenteric vein into the portal system.

Aetiology

The most common cause is arterial occlusion, usually of the superior mesenteric artery.

Classification:

- Thromboembolic arterial occlusion
- Mesenteric venous occlusion
- Systemic vasculitis
- Cardiovascular causes
- Secondary to intestinal obstruction
  - strangulated hernia
  - intussusception—usually in children

– volvulus—usually small bowel or sigmoid colon.

Clinical Features

The patient with an acute occlusion to their superior mesenteric artery may present with a sudden onset, severe colicky abdominal pain. The patient is classically elderly and has a past history of cardiac or arterial disease. Occasionally, the pain is vague and insidious.

Vomiting and diarrhoea can develop, and both may have a bloody element due to slow haemorrhage into the bowel lumen.

Physical signs are minimal initially and the patient is classically noted at this time to have pain out of proportion to the examination findings. However, as necrosis passes outwards from the mucosa, guarding, tenderness, abdominal distention and an absence of bowel sounds are apparent. **Shock is a late sign.**

Investigations

Patients with occlusion of the superior mesenteric artery may be investigated along the following lines:

- FBC: may show leucocytosis
- Biochemistry:
  – mildly raised serum amylase
  – increased inorganic phosphate indicates intestinal infarction
  – metabolic acidosis.
- Radiology:
  – plain abdominal X-ray:
    § absence of bowel gas at first
    § later, appearances of ileus, mucosal oedema and gas in the bowel wall and portal vein
  – mesenteric angiography:
  – often diagnostic, but difficult to do in the moribund patient.

Diagnosis

The diagnosis of occlusion of the superior mesenteric artery is often too late to save the patient's life. This is because the clinical presentation is often deceptive: signs are deceptively sparse and investigation is usually inconclusive at an early stage.

This condition should always be suspected in an arteriopath who develops unexplained abdominal pain. Prompt laparotomy to search for 'pale and pulseless' bowel is the best policy.

Treatment

The management of acute occlusion of the superior mesenteric artery may be divided into measures to stabilise the patient, and operative measures at laparotomy.

Aneurysmal Disease

An aneurysm is an abnormal, permanent, localised dilatation occurring in an artery or vein, or in the heart.

Arterial aneurysms of the abdominal aorta are most common and are most often due to atherosclerosis.

Classification of Aneurysms

Aneurysms may be true or false:

- A true aneurysm consists, at least in part, of the affected segment of blood vessel or, in the case of ventricular aneurysms, myocardium
- A false aneurysm is an aneurysm whose wall is formed from connective tissue which walls off a haematoma rather than from any part of the vessel wall or myocardium.

True aneurysms may be classified according to:

- Location
- Shape
- Aetiology.

Principles of Aneurysmal Surgery

Technique varies with respect to site. The principle aim is to correct the aneurysmal section of artery by a synthetic graft (often Dacron). Tube or bifurcation grafts are used for aorto-iliac and femoral aneurysms; autogenous saphenous vein grafts, for popliteal aneurysms.

Venous Diseases

This section, in addition to venous conditions requiring surgical treatment, contains deep venous thrombosis, which is a common post-operative problem.

Deep Vein Thrombosis

Deep vein thrombosis occurs in normal veins, usually the calf veins of the leg.

It is generally thought of as a complication of surgery or or illness. However, a number of situations predispose an individual to a deep vein thrombosis, and are encapsulated in Virchow's Triad.

The natural history is one of gradual breakdown of the thrombus with recanalisation.

Predisposing Factors

These may be classified according to Virchow's triad, although some have effects in more than one group.

Associated with changes in the vessel wall:

- Previous thrombo-embolism—the single most important risk factor
- Increasing age greater than 40 years old
- Smoking
- Local trauma
- Obesity.

Associated with increased blood coagulability:

- Malignancy e.g. thrombophlebitis migrans
- Pregnancy
- High dose oral contraceptive pills, oestrogen treatment

- Hormone replacement therapy
- Blood disorders:
  - polycythaemia
  - thrombocythaemia
  - congenital clotting disorders—deficiencies in protein C, protein S, anti-thrombin III
  - anti-phospholipid syndrome.

Associated with decreased blood flow:

- Surgery—complex systemic effects
- Immobility—e.g. debilitating illness, long distance travel
- Cardiac failure
- Dehydration.

Clinical Features

The classical features of DVT are noted in only half of cases, and include:

- Local swelling, tenderness and warmth
- Mild pyrexia
- Persistent tachycardia.

The exact presentation depends upon the site of thrombosis:

- Involving the calf-veins—calf swelling is usually modest. Homan's sign is positive but the test is not recommended because of the risk of pulmonary embolism.
- Involving the femoral vein—calf is swollen with local tenderness in the popliteal region or adductor canal.
- Involving the ilio-femoral veins—diffuse, and sometimes massive swelling of the entire lower limb. May progress to phlegmasia alba dolens, and in severe cases, to phlegmasia cerulia dolens.

When it occurs after an operation, the features of DVT are usually noted towards the end of the first post-operative week. They may occur earlier if the patient has been in hospital for some time pre-operatively. Careful scrutiny of the temperature chart and daily examination of the legs may predict impending thrombosis.

Investigations

Confirmation of suspected DVT may be made by:
- Venography—the definitive investigation but invasive
- Doppler ultrasound—good for ilio-femoral thrombosis.
- Impedance plethysmography
- Radio-iodine labelled fibrinogen uptake test
- D-dimers—this is not a diagnostic test, a raised level is suggestive, but not conclusive, evidence for a deep vein thrombosis.

Differential Diagnosis

This includes:
- Cellulitis
- Ruptured Baker's cyst
- Ruptured plantaris tendon—the patient may have heard it snap.

Management

Goals of treatment:
- Prevent pulmonary embolus
- Prevent severe post-thrombotic syndrome
- Prevent loss of limbs due to venous gangrene
- Alleviate symptoms.

The overriding consideration in the treatment of a DVT is the prevention of a potentially fatal pulmonary embolus. The main measure to achieve this is to prevent extension of the thrombus with anticoagulation, complemented by general maeasures.

Other more radical treatments such as thrombolysis and surgery are indicated when viability of the limb is threatened.

General Measures

The patient should be confined to bed for the first 24 hours with the foot of the bed elevated by 15-30 degrees. Pain and swelling should be alleviated by full length graduated compression stockings and analgesics. The patient should then be mobilised and encouraged to perform regular leg exercises.

Anticoagulation for Deep Venous Thrombosis

The standard treatment is for heparinasation of the patient and commencement on oral anticoagulant therapy. Heparinisation may be achieved via either use of intravenous heparin administration or subcutaneous administration of low molecular weight heparin:

- Intravenous heparin—in general, a loading dose of 5000 units is given, followed by 1000-1500 units per hour administered by continuous pump infusion. The activated partial thromboplastin time (APTT) is taken and the dose adjusted accordingly. Heparin anticoagulation is maintained until oral anticoagulation has achieved a target INR for treatment. Any major bleeding can be reversed with protamine sulphate, an effective heparin antedote.
- Subcutaneous low molecular weight heparin—this is used as alternative method of intravenous heparinisation in some centres; as with intravenous heparinisation, oral anticoagulation is commenced at the same time as heparinisation.

The dose of warfarin (or other oral anticoagulant) is adjusted according to the prothrombin time. Warfarin is generally continued for 3-6 months thus covering the period of greatest risk for thromboembolism and also preventing recurrence.

If there is a history of recurrent thromboembolism therapy may be continued indefinitely.

Thrombolysis for Deep Venous Thrombosis

Thrombolytic therapy uses plasminogen activating substances such as streptokinase, urokinase and alteplase to attempt to dissolve clots in the venous system.

It is only indicated in extensive thrombosis where it appears that the viability of the limb may be threatened i.e. in phlegmasia caerulia dolens. The thrombolytic agent is often delivered locally to the clot via a catheter since this may reduce the risk of haemorrhage due to systemic fibrinogenolysis.

The effectiveness of thrombolysis however is limited by the fact that peripheral thrombi are often old at presentation and furthermore thrombolysis does not appear to reduce the incidence of pulmonary emboli or post-thrombotic syndrome.

Surgery in Deep Venous Thrombosis

Thrombectomy is indicated when viability of the limb is threatened, as in phlegmasia cerulea dolens, particularly in situations where thrombolysis is contraindicated.

Surgery has also been recommended for iliofemoral thrombosis when it is felt that there is a particularly high risk of pulmonary embolism.

Thrombectomy is considered when the thrombus is non-adherent and less than 3 days old. It should always be followed by anticoagulation for 3-6 months.

The procedure is associated with further risk of thrombosis, haemorrhage and pulmonary embolism.

Varicose Veins

Varicose veins are dilated, tortuous veins in the leg.

Most varicose veins are primary; the remainder are secondary to other disorders such as deep venous thrombosis or pelvic occlusion.

Varicose veins occur in young adults and incidence increases with age to 80% at 60 years. Women are affected more frequently than men.

Varicose veins are asymptomatic in the majority of people, yet remain one of the most common reasons for surgical referral in the developed world.

Prominent varicosities usually develop slowly, over a period of 10-20 years. In most cases, the process begins in the groin with failure of the saphenofemoral valve.

The long saphenous system is involved in 90% of cases; the short system, in 10%.

Damage to the valves may produce deep venous incompetence.

Predisposing Factors

Congenital:

- Absence of valves in the iliac veins
- Abnormal vein wall elasticity
- Arteriovenous fistulae e.g. Robertson's giant limb.

Acquired:

- Obesity in women (but not in men)
- Prolonged standing
- Parity—women are affected six times more often than men, the majority of cases following a second or third pregnancy; important factors may include:
  - impaired venous return, due to pressure on the iliac veins from the pregnant uterus.
  - high level of progesterone which alters collagen structure, sometimes irreversibly, and relaxes smooth muscle.
- Previous deep vein thrombosis—valves damaged when the veins recanalise.

Pathogenesis

It is currently thought that the wall of the vein is weak in patients with varicose veins and that valvular incompentence follows rather than causes the dilatation of the vein.

This theory is supported by the observation that early dilatation is usually distal to an incompetent valve not proximal as might be expected if the damaged were caused by a descending valve incompetence.

Sites of Incompetent Valves

Incompetent valves commonly develop:

- In the groin, where the long saphenous vein joins the femoral vein.
- In the lower medial thigh, where the mid-thigh perforator joins the deep system at the adductor canal.
- Behind the knee, where the short saphenous vein joins the popliteal vein.
- Behind the medial border of the tibia, where several veins perforate the deep fascia of the calf.

Investigations

Ideally all patients with varicose veins would have colour duplex ultrasound scanning to determine the characteristics of blood flow in the leg. Unfortunately this is not possible and so duplex scanning is reserved for the following groups of patients with:

- Recurrent varicose veins
- A history of superficial thrombophlebitis
- A history of DVT
- Varicose eczema
- Haemosiderin discolouration
- Lipodematosclerosis
- Venous ulceration.

Clinical Features

Symptoms commonly associated with varicose veins are:

- Disfigurement:
  - Patients are frequently disturbed by the poor cosmetic appearance of their legs
  - both their concern and their symptoms may worsen in the summer when the legs are warm and exposed.
- Pain:
  - legs frequently ache, especially after prolonged standing

  - patients often describe a dull, heavy, "burning" sensation that becomes more severe as the day progresses
  - in women, symptoms may worsen in the few days prior to menstruation.
- Itching:
  - the skin over the varices may itch
  - may be associated with varicose eczema
- Heaviness
- Worry:
  - patients may present because of concern about possible complications such as ulceration.

Examination:
- Varices appear on standing and disappear when Recumbent
- Positive Brodie-Trendelenburg test
- Doppler flow studies identify 'backflow' through incompetent valves.

Management

Treatment of varicose veins may be indicated to relieve discomfort, to prevent or ameliorate complications, or for cosmetic reasons.

Methods:
- Conservative
- Surgical:
  - sclerotherapy—permanent obliteration of varices
  - open operation—removal of varices with ligation of incompetent perforaters

About one-third of cases can be managed by offering common sense advice as to how to take care for their legs.

Conservative

The aim is to improve venous return and reduce pressure in varicose superficial veins. It should be considered in:

- Patient's with uncomplicated varicosities
- The pregnant, the elderly or the unfit
- Patient's who refuse other forms of treatment.

Methods include:

- Encourage walking
- Discourage prolonged sitting or standing
- Keep legs elevated when sitting to increase venous return
- Lose weight, if appropriate
- Wear supporting elastic stockings which compress superficial veins and prevent reflux from deep veins:
  - the stockings should extend from the distal metatarsals to just below the knee
  - avoid extending to the thigh unless they can be secured by means of a garter
  - use carefully because of potential tourniquet effect.

Sclerotherapy (varicose leg veins)

Injection sclerotherapy is indicated for small, disfiguring varicose veins below the knee. It is done as an outpatient procedure.

The affected veins are injected with a sclerosant such as 1-3% sodium tetradecyl sulphate. Compressive bandages are worn for 1-6 weeks to enable fibrosis to occur. Recurrences are treated by further injections.

Injection sclerotherapy is not advised:

- For major varicosities, particularly in the thigh, because of the danger of causing thrombosis in femoral or popliteal deep veins
- In patient's with acute infective thrombophlebitis or a pre-existing deep thrombus
- In women who are pregnant or taking the combined oral contraceptive pill.

Surgery

Open operation is recommended when the primary site of incompetence is in the long or short saphenous veins. The affected veins are removed and their associated incompetent perforators ligated or avulsed.

Prior to surgery, the affected veins must be marked since they will not be visible during operation with the patient recumbent. Low-dose subcutaneous heparin should be offered to any patient with a history of superficial or deep venous thrombosis, or with other risk factors for deep venous thrombosis.

Often, the long saphenous vein must be removed. It is exposed in the groin and it's tributaries ligated at the sapheno-femoral junction. An intraluminal stripper is passed and the vein removed.

Increasingly modern practice is to preserve the long saphenous vein when possible, unless extensively dilated because of it's possible use in coronary artery bypass grafting.

Individual varices below the knee may be avulsed through small skin incisions over the veins.

The legs are bandaged at the end of the procedure, and though practise varies bandages or compression stockings remain in place for 1-2 weeks. The patient is encouraged to exercise daily after the first 24 hours and to keep the limb elevated when sitting.

Recurrence after operation is most frequently caused by failure to ligate all the tributaries of the long saphenous vein in the groin.

Clinical Priority

The following approach to prioritising surgery for varicose veins has been proposed:

- Top priority for varicose veins with complications
- Medium priority for cases of trunk varicosities
- Low priority for reticular varicosities and telangiectasiae.

Chapter 10

Pediatrics Surgery

INTRODUCTION

Neonatal Physiologic Characteristics

Water Metabolism

Water represents is distributed into extracellular fluid (ECF) and intracellular fluid (ICF) compartment. The 70 to 80% of the body weight of the normal neonate and premature baby respectively. TBW ECF compartment is one-third the TBW with sodium as principal cation, and chloride and bicarbonate as anions.The ICF compartment is two-third the TBW with potassium the principal cation. The Newborn's metabolic rate is high and extra energy is needed for maintenance of body temperature and growth. A change in body water occurs upon entrance of the fetus to his new extrauterine existence. There is a gradual decrease in body water and the extracellular fluid compartment with a concomitant increase in the intracellular fluid compartment. This shift is interrupted with a premature birth. The newborn's body surface area is relatively much greater than theadults and heat loss is a major factor. Insensible water loss are from the lung (1/3) and skin (2/3).Transepithelial (skin) water is the major component and decreases with increase in post-natal age. Insensible water loss is affected by gestational age, body temperature (radiant warmers), and phototherapy Neonatal renal function is generally adequate to meet the needs of the normal full-term infant but may be limited during periods of stress. Renal characteristics of newborns are a low glomerular filtration rate and concentration ability (limited urea in medullary interticium) which makes them less tolerant to dehydration. The neonate is metabolically active and production of solute to excrete in the urine is high. The kidney in the newborn can only concentrate to about 400 mOsm/L initially (500-600 mOsm/L the full-term compared to 1200mOsm/L for an adult), and therefore requires 2-4 cc/kg/hr urine production to clear the renal solute load. The older child needs about 1-2 cc/kg/hr and the adult 0.5-1 cc/kg/hr.

Metabolic and Host Defenses

Handling of the breakdown products of hemoglobin is also a difficult task for the premature infant. The ability of the immature liver to conjugate bilirubin is reduced, the life span of the red blood cell is short, and the bilirubin load presented to the circulation via the enterohepatic route is increased. "Physiologic" jaundice is,therefore, higher in the preterm infant and persists for a longer period. Unfortunately, the immature brain has an increased susceptibility to the neurotoxic effects of high levels of unconjugated bilirubin, and kernicterus can develop in the preterm baby at a relatively low level of bilirubin. Infant produce heat by increasing metabolic activity and using brown fat. Below the 35°C the newborn experiences lassitude, depressed respiration, bradycardia, metabolic acidosis, hypoglycemia, hyperkalemia, elevated BUN and oliguria (neonatal cold injury syndrome). Factors that precipitate further these problems are: prematurity, prolonged surgery, and eviscerated bowel (gastroschisis).

Surgical Response of Newborns

The endocrine and metabolic response to surgical stress in newborns is characterized by catabolic metabolism. An initial elevation in cathecolamines, cortisol and endorphins upon stimulation by noxious stimuli occurs; a defense mechanism of the organism to mobilize stored energy reserves, form new ones and start cellular catabolism. Cortisol circadian responsiveness during the first week of life is diminished, due to inmaturation of the adrenal gland. Cortisol is responsible for protein breakdown, release of gluconeogenic amino acids from muscle, and fat lipolysis with release of fatty acids. Glucagon secretion is increased. Plasma insulin increase is a reflex to the hyperglycemic effect, although a resistance to its anabolic function is present.

HEAD AND NECK LESIONS

Thyroglossal Duct Cysts

Thyroglossal duct cyst (TDC) is the **most common congenital anterior midline neck mass** usually (2/3of cases) presenting before the second decade of life. Symptoms appear at an average age of four with the sudden appearance of a cystic mass at the angle of neck level moving with tongue protrusion and swallowing. Males are more commonly affected than females. TDC is an embryologic anomaly arising from epithelial remnant left after descent of the eveloping thyroid from the foramen cecum. The lining is cuboidal, columnar or pseudostratified epithelium. TDC is associated to discomfort, infection and a slight probability of malignancy. A legally protective requirement is to document that the mass is not ectopic thyroid gland. Diagnosis is physical. Sonograms will show a cyst between 0.4 and 4 cm in diameter, with variable sonographic appearance and no correlation with pathological findings of infection or inflammation. Once infected surgical excision is more difficult and recurrence will increase. Management is Sistrunk's operation: Excision of cyst with resection of duct along with the central portion of hyoid bone (a minimum of 10-15 mm of hyoid bone should be removed) and some muscle surrounding the proximal ductules (the length of single duct above the hyoid bone spreads into many ductuli as it approach the foramen cecum). Extensive dissection can cause pharyngodynia. The greatest opportunity for cure is surgery at initial non-inflamed presentation. Inadequate excision is a risk factor for further recurrence.

Cystic Hygroma

Cystic hygroma (CH) is an uncommon congenital lesion of the lymphatic system appearing as a multilocular fluid filled cavity most commonly in the back neck region, occasionally associated with extensive involvement of airway or vital structures. The etiology is intrauterine failure of lymphatics to communicate with the venous system. Prenatal diagnosis can be done during the first trimester of pregnancy as a huge neck tumor. Differential diagnosis includes teratomas, encephalocele, hemangiomas, etc. There is a strong correlation between prenatal dx and Turner's syndrome (> 50%), structural defects (Noonan's syndrome) and chromosomic anomalies (13, 18, 21). Early diagnosis (< 30 wk gestation) is commonly associated to those anomalies, non-immune hydrops and dismal outcome (fetal death). Spontaneous regression is less likely but can explain webbed neck of Turner and Noonan's children. Prenatal dx should be followed by cytogenetic analysis: chorionic villous sampling, amniocentesis, or nuchal fluid cell obtained from the CH itself to determine fetal karyotype and provide counseling of pregnancy. Late diagnosis (>30 wks) should be delivered in tertiary center prepare to deal with dystocia and postnatal dyspnea of newborn. The airway should be secured before cord clamping in huge lesions. Intracystic injection of OK432 (lyophilized product of Streptococcus pyogenes) caused cystic (hygromas) lymphangiomas to become inflamed and led to subsequent cure of the lesion without side effects.

Cat Scratch Disease

Cat Scratch Disease (CSD) is a self-limited condition transmitted by a Bartonella species (Rochalimaea henselae) present in unaffected kitten paws. Following inoculation by a scratch and one to two weeks of incubation period, malaise, fever, headache, anorexia and swelling of the regional lymph nodes follow. The adenopathy generally develops in the upper extremity (epitrochlear, axilla) or head/neck areas, is minimally tender and can develop fluctuation. Median age is 14 years with highest attack rate in children less than ten years of age. The diagnosis relies on the presence of symptoms, signs, physical exam (characteristic papule at the site of the scratch), history of exposure to a cat, and a positive immunofluorescent assay for Bartonella antibodies. Most patients with clinically diagnosed CSD developed an immunologic response to Bartonella species. Conservative symptomatic management is recommended for most children since the node will eventually disappear spontaneously. In other cases' aspiration of fluctuant nodes is alleviating. Antibiotics are recommended during severe cases. Overall prognosis is good.

INTESTINAL OBSTRUCTION IN A NEWBORN

Signs and Symptoms

1. Bilious vomiting is always abnormal.
2. Abdominal distention (scaphoid abdomen possible).
3. Delayed, scanty or no passage of meconium.
4. Polyhydramnios in mother.
5. Down's syndrome
6. Family history
   a. Hirschsprung's disease
   b. Diabetic mother
   c. Jejunal atresia

Work-up (Logical approach)

1. While the infant is being studied, it must be kept in mind that the problem may be "non-surgical".

a. Sepsis of the newborn with associated ileus is the most important cause of non-surgical bilious vomiting and abdominal distention.
b. Intracranial lesions
   i. Hydrocephalus
   ii. Subdural hemorrhage.
c. Renal disease associated with uremia.
   i. Renal agenesis
   ii. Polycystic disease
   iii. Other urinary tract anomalies which may be associated with severe hydronephrosis.

2. Plain roentgenograms of the abdomen.
   a. Diagnostic in complete high intestinal obstruction-no gas in distal small bowel.
      i. Double bubble in duodenal obstruction.
      ii. Few gas filled loops beyond duodenum indicates jejunal atresia.
   b. Many gas filled loops (requires 24 hours) indicates some form of low intestinal obstruction.
      i. Ileal atresia
      ii. Meconium ileus(an unfortunate misnomer)-obstruction of the distal small intestine by thick undigested meconium.
      iii. Meconium plug syndrome-obstruction of colon by a plug of meconium.
      iv. Small left colon syndrome.
      v. Hirschsprung's disease-congenital aganglionosis of colon starting with the rectum.
      vi. Colonic atresia.
   c. May be nonspecific in instances of malrotation of the intestines. This diagnosis must always be considered in neonates with unexplained bilious vomiting.
   d. Calcifications-at some time during fetal life meconium was (is) present in the abdomen.
3. Contrast enema will differentiate the various types of low intestinal obstruction.
   a. Microcolon-complete obstruction of the small bowel.

b. Meconium plug syndrome-colon dilated proximal to an intraluminal mass.
c. Hirschsprung's disease-although it may appear to be diagnostic, not reliable in the newborn.
d. Small left colon syndrome-colon dilated to the splenic flexure, then becomes narrow.

4. Upper G.I.- the procedure of choice in diagnosing malrotation of the intestines. In the past a contrast enema was thought to be the diagnostic test of choice in instances of malrotation but the cecum and ascending colon can be in normal position in an infant or child with malrotation of the intestines.
5. Rectal biopsy- a pathologist competent in reading the slides is essential and should not be taken for granted.
   a. Suction biopsy of the rectal mucosa and submucosa- best screening procedure to rule out Hirschsprung's disease (ganglion cells are present in the submucosa), and is diagnostic in experienced hands.
   b. Full thickness biopsy of the rectal wall may be necessary if the suction biopsy is non-diagnostic or if the pathologist is unwilling or unable to make the diagnosis of aganglionosis on a suction biopsy specimen.
   This procedure is difficult in the small infant and has been replaced by the suction biopsy in most centers.
   c. All newborns who have delayed passage of meconium associated with a suspicious contrast enema should have a suction biopsy of the rectal mucosa and submucosa. With this technique, Hirschsprung's disease will be diagnosed early before it is complicated with enterocolitis. If delayed passage of meconium is "cured" by rectal stimulation(suppository, thermometer, or finger), it must be kept in mind that the diagnosis of Hirschsprung's disease is still a possibility. Whether or not a suction biopsy of the rectum is done before the infant goes home depends

on the clinical setting but the safe course of action is to do the rectal biopsy before discharge. Parents may not call before the infant gets into trouble with enterocolitis.

d. Suction biopsy of the rectum is probably indicated in all cases of so called meconium plug syndrome or small left colon syndrome. If the suction biopsy is not done, the infant must be observed for recurrent gastrointestinal symptoms. A breast-fed infant who has Hirschsprung's disease can "get by" for a prolonged period of time.

Esophageal Atresia a/o Tracheo-esophageal fistula

The trachea and esophagus initially begin as a ventral diverticulum of the foregut during the third intrauterine week of life. A proliferation of endodermal cells appears on the lateral aspect of this growing diverticulum. These cell masses will divide the foregut into trachea and esophageal tubes. Whether interruption of this normal event leads to tracheo-esophageal anomalies, or during tracheal growth atresia of the esophagus results because of fistulous fixation of the esophagus to the trachea remnant to be proven.

Classification

EA with distal TEF (87%)- the most common anomaly, the NG tube coiled at T4-5 level and gas will be seen in the KUB. EA without TEF (8%) - pure esophageal atresia, NG coiled at T4-5 level with airless abdomen. TEF without atresia (4%) - pure tracheo-esophageal fistula. EA with proximal TEF (<1%). EA with proximal and distal TEF (<1%) Congenital isolated tracheo-esophageal fistula (TEF) occurs as 4-6% of the disorders of the esophagus bringing problems during early diagnosis and management. More than H-type is N-type, due to the obliquity of the fistula from trachea (carina or main bronchi) to esophageal side (see the figure) anatomically at the level of the neck root (C7-T1). Pressure changes between both structure can cause entrance of air into the esophagus, or esophageal content into the trachea. Thus, the clinical manifestation that we must be aware for early diagnosis are: cyanosis, coughing and choking with feedings, recurrent chest infections, persistent gastrointestinal distension with air, and hypersalivation. Diagnosis is confirmed with a well-done esophagogram, or video-esophagogram (high success rates, establish level of the TEF). Barium in the trachea could be caused by aspiration during the procedure. Upon radiologic doubt bronchoscopy should be the next diagnostic step. Any delay in surgery is generally due to delay in diagnosis rather than delay in presentation. Management consists of surgical closure of the TEF through a right cervical approach. Hint: a small guide-wire threaded through the fistula during bronchoscopy may be of some help. Working in the tracheo-esophageal groove can cause injury to the recurrent laryngeal nerve with vocal cord paralysis. Recurrence after closure is rare.

Diagnostic Characteristics

The incidence is one in every 2500 live births. The mother might show polyhydramnios since the fetus is unable to swallow amniotic fluid. (May be responsible for early delivery). Polyhydramnios is most commonly seen in pure esophageal atresia type. Choking, coughing and regurgitation with first feed. Excessive salivation, cyanosis with feedings. Inability to pass feeding tube into the stomach. Contrast studies (UGIS, esophagogram) are rarely needed, and of potential disaster (aspiration of contrast material). Abdominal films should be obtained to rule out the occurrence of associated gastrointestinal anomalies. Isolated TEF is more difficult to diagnose and may require repeated lateral esophagograms, bronchoscopy and esophagoscopy. **Management**

Correct dehydration, acid-base disturbances, respiratory distress and decompress proximal esophageal pouch (Replogle tube). Evaluate for associated conditions such as **VACTERL** association (3 or more):

- **V**ertebral anomalies i.e. hemivertebrae, spina bifida
- **A**nal malformations i.e. imperforate anus
- **C**ardiac malformations i.e. VSD, ASD, Tetralogy Fallot
- **T**racheo-**E**sophageal fistula (must be one of the associated conditions)
- **R**enal deformities i.e. absent kidney, hypospadia, etc.
- **L**imb dysplasia.

Early surgical repair (transpleural or extrapleural) for those babies with no evidence of pneumonia, adequate weight (>1200 gm) and no significant associated anomalies. Babies with Chest-X-Ray positive findings, but adequate ABG's can also be primarily repaired. Delayed repair (gastrostomy first) for all other patients. Surgical repair consist of a 4th intercostal space right muscle-sparing thoracotomy (side of thoracotomy is contralateral to side of aortic arch of patient), closure of tracheo-esophageal fistula and primary esophago-esophagostomy. Esophagogram is done 7-10 days after repair. Complications after surgery are: Anastomotic leak, anastomotic stricture, gastroesophageal reflux, tracheomalacia, and recurrent TEF. The three most common anastomotic complications are in order of frequency: stricture, leakage and recurrent TEF. Recurrent TEF after surgical repair for esophageal atresia occurs in approximately 3-15% of cases. Tension on the anastomoses followed by leakage may lead to local inflammation with breakage of both suture lines enhancing the chance of recurrent TEF. Once established, the fistula allows saliva and food into the trachea, hence clinical suspicion of this diagnosis arises with recurrent respiratory symptoms associated with feedings after repair of esophageal atresia. Diagnosis is confirmed with cineradiography of the esophagus or bronchoscopy. A second thoracotomy is very hazardous, but has proved to be the most effective method to close the recurrent TEF. Either a pleural or pericardial flap will effectively isolate the suture line. Pericardial flap is easier to mobilize, provides sufficient tissue to use and serves as template for ingrowth of new mucosa should leakage occur. Other alternatives are endoscopic diathermy obliteration, laser coagulation, or fibrin glue deposition.

Achalasia

Achalasia in children is an uncommon esophageal motor disorder distinguished by clinical, radiological and manometrics features. Incidence is estimated in 0.1 cases/year per 100,000 population under 14 years of age. Clinical presentation is characterized by progressive dysphagia, regurgitation, weight loss, chest pain and nocturnal cough. Infants exhibit failure to thrive. Diagnosis is established by barium swallow and confirmed by manometry and motility studies. Ba swallow shows' esophageal dilatation, motility alteration and a small caliber (**bird-beak**) cardio-esophageal junction. Manometry reveals elevated E-G sphincter pressure, non- peristaltic esophageal contraction and failed relaxation of lower esophageal sphincter upon swallowing. Videofluoroscopy can be of help in the screening of esophageal motors disorders. Esophageal pneumatic balloon dilatation is not an effective method of treatment in children due to the high rate of recurrence of symptoms. Primary therapy is surgical (Heller's modified esophagomyotomy), and results are similar after a transabdominal or thoracic approach. Many authors favor a concomitant antireflux procedures in these patients. Nifedipine can be of help as a short management in preparation for surgery. Long-term result presents' a connection between achalasia and malignant disease of the esophagus.

Gastro-duodenal Anomalies

1. *Gastric Anomalies:* Congenital gastric outlet obstruction is extremely rare. It occurs either in

the pyloric or antral region. Antral membranes (web or diaphragm) are thin, soft and pliable, composed of mucosa/submucosa, and located eccentric 1-3 cm proximal to pyloro-duodenal junction. They probably represent the developmental product of excess local endodermal proliferation and redundancy. The diagnosis should rely on history, contrast roentgenology studies and endoscopic findings. Symptoms are those of recurrent non-bilious vomiting and vary according to the diameter of aperture of the membrane. There is a slight male predominance with fair distribution between age groups in children. Associated conditions: pyloric stenosis, peptic ulcer and cardiac. History of polyhydramnios in the mother. Demonstration of a radiolucent line perpendicular to the long axis of the antrum is diagnostic of a web. Endoscopy corroborates the diagnosis. Management can be either surgical or non-surgical. Surgical Tx is successful in symptomatic pt. and consist of pyloroplasty with incision or excision of the membrane. Other alternative is endoscopic balloon dilatation or transection of the web. Non-obstructive webs found incidentally can be managed medically with small curd formula and antispasmodics. The presence of an abnormally dilated gastric bubble in prenatal sonography should alert the physician toward the diagnosis of congenital antro-pyloric obstruction.

2. *Pyloric Stenosis:* Is an abnormality of the pyloric musculature (hypertrophy) causing gastric outlet obstruction in early infancy. The incidence is 3 per 1000 live births. The etiology is unknown, but pylorospasm to formula protein cause a work hypertrophy of the muscle. Diagnostic characteristics are: non-bilious projectile vomiting classically 3-6 weeks of age, palpable pyloric muscle "olive", contrast studies are not necessary when the pyloric muscle is palpated, enlarged width and length in ultrasonography. The treatment consist in correction of hypochloremic alkalosis and state of

dehydration and performing a Fredet-Ramstedt modified pyloromyotomy. Post-operative management consist of: 50% will have one to several episodes of vomiting, usually can feed and go home in 24-36 hours, initial feeds start 8-12 hours after surgery.

3. *Duodenal Malformations:* Can be intrinsic (Atresia, Stenosis, Webs) or extrinsic (Annular pancreas, Ladd's bands). Occur distal or proximal to the ampulla of Vater. Most commonly distal to ampulla and therefore bilious vomiting is present. (Note: Bilious vomiting is surgical until proven otherwise in a baby).

   "Windsock" webs have clinical importance because of their tendency to be confused with distal duodenal obstruction and because of the frequent occurrence of an anomalous biliary duct entering along their medial margin.

   Embryology: The first major event in the differentiation of the duodenum, hepatobiliary tree, and pancreas occurs at about the third week in gestation, when the biliary and pancreatic buds form at the junction of the foregut and the midgut. The duodenum at this time is a solid cord of epithelium, which undergoes vacuolization followed by recanalization and restitution of the intestinal lumen over 3-4 weeks of normal development. Failure of recanalization of the second part of the duodenum results in congenital obstruction of the lumen, often in conjunction with developmental malformation of the pancreatic anlagen and the terminal part of the biliary tree. In support of this concept is the high incidence of annular pancreas observed, believed to represent a persistence of the ventral pancreatic anlage in association with intrinsic duodenal obstruction.

The diagnostic characteristics are: bilious vomiting, history of polyhydramnios in mother, KUB with classic "Double-bubble" appearance, a microcolon in barium enema study or malrotation. Treatment consist in:

1. duodeno-duodenostomy bypass for atresias, annular pancreas, and some stenosis.
2. duodenoplasty for webs, and stenosis, and
3. lysis of Ladd's bands and Ladd's procedure for malrotation.

Associated anomalies are: Down's syndrome (20-30%), VACTERL syndrome, CNS anomalies and cardiac anomalies.

Malrotation and Volvulus

Embryology: The rotation and normal fixation of the intestinal tract takes place within the first three months of fetal life. In the earliest stages when the intestinal tract is recognizable as a continuous tube, the stomach, small intestine, and colon constitute a single tube with its blood supply arising posteriorly. The midgut portion of this tube, from the second portion of the duodenum to the mid-transverse colon, lengthens and migrates out into an extension of the abdomen, which lies at the base of the umbilical cord. Here this loop of bowel undergoes a 270-degree counterclockwise twist at its neck. In the center of the twisted loop lie the blood vessels that will become the superior mesenteric artery and vein. After rotation, the small intestine quite rapidly withdraws into the abdominal cavity, with the duodenum and the proximal jejunum going first. During this process the duodenojejunal junction goes beneath and to the left of the base of the superior mesenteric vessels. This leaves the upper intestine, including the stomach and the duodenum, encircling the superior mesenteric vessels like a horseshoe with its opening on the left side of the embryo. The small intestine then follows into the abdomen, and withdrawal of the right half of the colon takes place so that it lies to the left. At the next step, the cecum and the right colon begin to travel across the top of the superior mesenteric vessels and then down to the right lower quadrant. The colon now lies draped across the top of the superior mesenteric vessels, again like a horseshoe, with its opening placed inferiorly. The duodenojejunal loop is said to attach to the posterior abdominal wall soon after its turn, whereas the mesenteric attachments of the entire colon and of the remaining small bowel gradually adhere after they arrive in their normal positions. In malrotation the right colon can create peritoneal attachments that include and obstruct the third portion of the duodenum (Ladd's bands).

The diagnostic hallmarks are: bilious vomiting (the deadly vomit), abdominal distension and metabolic acidosis. A UGIS is more reliable than barium enema, most patients present in first month of life (neonatal), but may present at any time.

The treatment is immediate operation; volvulus often means strangulation. Needs fluid and electrolyte replacement. Ladd's procedure consist of: reduce volvulus with a counterclockwise rotation, place small bowel in right abdomen, lysed Ladd's bands, place large bowel in left abdomen, do an appendectomy. In cases of questionable non-viable bowel a second look procedure is required. Failure to make early diagnosis and operate may lead to dead midgut with resultant short bowel syndrome.

Intestinal Atresias

Intestinal atresias are the product of a late intrauterine mesenteric vascular accident (blood supply was not received by a portion of bowel) as attested by Louw and Barnard in 1955. They are equally distributed from the ligament of Treitz to the ileocecal junction. Colonic atresias are very rare. There is proximal bowel dilatation, with distal (unused) micro-bowel. The diagnosis is suspected with maternal history of polyhydramnios (the higher the atresia), bilious vomiting, abdominal distension and obstipation. KUB shows "thumb-size" dilated bowel loops, and barium enema a microcolon of disuse. Louw classified them into:

Type I: an intraluminal diaphragm with seromuscular continuity.

Type II: cord-like segment between the bowel blinds ends.

Type IIIA: atresia with complete separation of blind ends and V-shaped mesenteric defect (see figure), the most commonly found.

Type IIIB: jejunal atresia with extensive mesenteric defect and distal ileum acquiring its blood supply entirely from a single ileocolic artery. The distal bowel coils itself around the vessel, giving the appearance of an "apple peel"deformity. **Type IV:** multiple atresias of the small intestine.

After preoperative stabilization (GI decompression, electrolytes disturbances' correction, antibiotherapy, and normothermia), treatment consists of exploratory laparotomy, resection of proximal dilated intestine, and end to oblique anastomosis in distal jejuno-ileal atresias. Tapering jejunoplasty with anastomosis is preferred in proximal defects.

Meconium Ileus

Meconium ileus is a neonatal intraluminal intestinal obstruction caused by inspissated meconium blocking the distal ileum. Occurs in 10-15% of all patients with cystic fibrosis, and 85-95% of patients with meconium ileus have cystic fibrosis. The meconium has a reduced water, abnormal high protein and mucoprotein content, the result of decreased pancreatic enzyme activity and prolonged small bowel intestinal transit time.

Meconium Ileus is classified into two types: **(1) Simple meconium ileus**: The distal small bowel (10-30 cm of distal ileum) is relatively small, measuring less than 2 cm in diameter and contains concretions of gray, inspissated meconium with the consistency of thick glue or putty. It is often beaklike in appearance, conforming to the shape of the contained pellets. Proximally, the mid-ileum is large, measuring up to 7 cm in diameter. It is greatly distended by a mass of extremely thick, tenacious, dark green or tarry meconium. The unused small colon (microcolon) contains a small amount of inspissated mucus or grayish meconium. **(2) Complicated meconium ileus**: usually occurs during the prenatal period associated to volvulus, atresias, gangrene, perforation or peritonitis. A cystic mass or atresia of the bowel may occur. The degree of obstruction varies, may be cured in mild cases by rectal irrigations. Failure to pass meconium, abdominal distension and vomiting are seen in more severe cases. The diagnosis is suspected with findings of: multiple loops of dilated small bowel and coarse granular **"soap-bubble" appearance** on plain abdominal films. Some cases may show calcifications in the peritoneum (Meconium peritonitis). The Sweat Testis diagnostic of cystic fibrosis (value over 60 meq/L of sweat sodium or chloride are diagnostic). This test is not useful in infant during first weeks of life.

Therapy is either: (1) Nonoperative- should be tried first. It consist of a careful gastrografin enema after the baby is well-hydrated. Gastrografin is a hyperosmolar aqueous solution of meglumine diatrizoate containing 0.1% polysorbate-80 (tween-80, a wetting agent) and 37% iodine. Its success is due to the high osmolarity (1700 mOsm/liter) which draws fluid into the bowel and softens and loosens the meconium. (2) Surgical therapy that has included: ileostomy with irrigation, resection with anastomosis, and resection with ileostomy (Mikulicz, Bishop-Kopp, and Santulli). Post-operative management includes: 10% acetylcysteine p.o., oral feedings (Pregestimil), pancreatic enzyme replacement, and prophylactic pulmonary therapy. Long-term prognosis depends on the degree of severity and progression of cystic fibrosis pulmonary disease.

Hirschsprung's Disease

Hirschsprung's is the congenital absence of parasympathetic innervation of the distal intestine. The colon proximal to the aganglionic segment, in an effort to overcome the partial obstruction, becomes distended and its wall markedly thickened because of muscle hypertrophy. Occurs 1 in 1000-1500 live births with a 4:1 male predominance.

The parasympathetic ganglion cell network located between the circular and longitudinal muscle layersis referred to as Auerbach's plexus, whereas Meissner's plexus is the submucosal layer of ganglion cells just beneath the muscularis mucosa. In Hirschsprung's disease, ganglion cells are absent from all layers. That aganglionic segment usually involves the terminal intestine, i.e. the rectum or rectosigmoid. The aganglionic segment may, however, include the entire large bowel and even small bowel. Hirschsprung's disease (HD) is characterized by lack of enteric ganglion cells, hyperplasia of abnormal nerve fibers and a non-propulsive, non-relaxing segment of bowel. Classically the etiology is attributed to a failure of cranio-caudal migration of parasympathetic neural crest cells to the distal bowel. A plausible explanation for the failure of relaxation of the bowel involved is a deficiency of enteric inhibitory nerves that mediates the relaxation phase of peristalsis. This nerves are intrinsic to the gut and are classify as nonadrenergic and non-cholinergic. Nitric oxide (NO) has recently been implicated as the neurotransmitter which mediates the relaxation of smooth muscle of the GI tract in HD. It's absence in aganglionic bowel might account for the failure of relaxation during peristalsis. Besides, adhesions molecules (absent in aganglionic bowel) during early embryogenesis might restrict the neuro-ectodermal origin involved in the initial contact between nerves and muscle cell (synaptogenesis) suggesting that developmental anomaly of innervated muscle and absent NO causes the spasticity characteristic of HD.

Symptoms usually begin at birth, frequently with delayed passage of meconium. Any newborn who fails to pass meconium in the first 24-48 hours of life should be evaluated for possible Hirschsprung's disease. In some infants, the presentation is that of complete intestinal obstruction. Others have relatively few symptoms until several weeks of age, when the classic symptom of constipation has its onset. Diarrhea is not uncommon but differs from the usual infantile diarrhea in that it is associated with abdominal distension. Occasionally the patient will go many years with mild constipation and diagnosis will be delayed. The diagnosis is first suspected based on history and physical examinations (characteristically there is no stool in rectum and abdominal distension is painless). Initial evaluation includes an unprepared barium enema (the first enema should be a barium enema!). The aganglionic rectum appears of normal caliber or spastic, there is a transition zone and then dilated colon proximal to the aganglionic segment. 24-hrs delayed films shows poor emptying with barium throughout the colon, as opposed to the child with psychogenic stool holding in whom the barium generally collects in the distal rectosigmoid. Rectal suction biopsy is then performed. This can be done without anesthesia and the submucosal plexus is examined for ganglion cells. With experience, a good pathologist (should be an expert!), can identify the presence or absence of ganglion cells in this specimen without a full thickness biopsy. Difficulty in interpreting the specimen or not enough to include several slides of submucosa would require a full-thickness biopsy for definitive diagnosis generally done under general anesthesia. Some centers employ manometry, histochemical studies or special stains for diagnosis. These special studies are only as good as the person performing them and interpreting the results. The initial treatment requires performing a "leveling" colostomy in the most distal colon with ganglion cells present. This requires exploration with multiple seromuscular biopsies of the colon wall to determine the exact extend of the aganglionosis. The colostomy is placed above the transition zone. Placement of the colostomy in an area of aganglionosis will lead to persistent obstruction. Once the child has reached an adequate size and age (6-12 months; 20 pounds or more), a formal pull-through procedure is done. Some of this are: Swenson, Duhamel and Soave procedures. Current preference is for Soave procedure (modified endorectal pull-through) . Recently a laparoscopic pull-through procedure avoiding the colostomy is being used in early life with promising results.

Imperforate Anus

Embryology- Between 4-6 weeks, the cloaca becomes the common depository for the developing urinary, genital and rectal systems. The cloaca is quite promptly divided into an anterior urogenital sinus and a posterior intestinal canal by the urorectal septum. Two lateral folds of cloacal tissue join the urorectal septum to complete the separation of the urinary and rectal tracts.

Diagnostic evaluation include physical exam for clues such as: meconium "pearls", bucket handle anus, a fistula or meconium at meatus (urethra). Radiography could be of help initially by using Wangensteen-Rice "upside-down" film with opaque marker, sacral films, urogram (IVP and cystourethrogram). Through the distal stoma of the initial colostomy a contrast study (colostogram) can be done to further delineate the recto-urethral fistula associated.

Associated Anomalies: (i) Gastrointestinal- 10-20% of patients with imperforate anus have another GI lesion such as esophageal atresia, intestinal atresia or malrotation. (ii) Cardiovascular- approximately 7% have associated CV lesions. (iii) Skeletal- approximately 6% have skeletal lesions such as spina bifida or agenesis of the sacrum. (iv) Genitourinary- 25-40% of patients will have associated genitourinary anomalies. The incidence is higher with supralevator lesions than with infralevator lesions. The repair has been revolutionize by Peña approach (Posterior sagittal anorectoplasty procedure). The most important decision in the initial management of Imperforate Anus (IA) male patient during the neonatal period is whether the baby needs a colostomy and/or another kind of urinary diversion procedure to prevent sepsis or metabolic derangements. Male patients will benefit from perineal inspection to check for the presence of a fistula (wait 16-24 hours of life before deciding). During this time start antibiotherapy, decompress the GI tract, do a urinalysis to check for meconium cells, and an ultrasound of abdomen to identify urological associated anomalies. Perineal signs in low malformations that will NOT need a colostomy are: meconium in perineum, bucket-handle defect, anal membrane and anal stenosis. These infants can be managed with a perineal anoplasty during the neonatal period with an excellent prognosis. Meconium in urine shows the pt has a fistula between the rectum and the urinary tract. Flat "bottom" or perineum (lack of intergluteal fold), and absence of anal dimple indicates poor muscles and a rather high malformation needing a colostomy. Patients with no clinical signs at 24 hours of birth will need a invertogram or cross-table lateral film in prone position to decide rectal pouch position. Bowel > 1 cm from skin level will need a colostomy, and bowel < 1 cm from skin can be approach perineally. Those cases with high defect are initially managed with a totally diverting colostomy. Diverting the fecal stream reduces the chances of genito-urinary tract contamination and future damage.

The most frequent defect in females patient with imperforate anus (IA) is vestibular fistula, followed by vaginal fistulas. In more than 90% of females cases perineal inspection will confirmed the diagnosis. These infants require a colostomy before final corrective surgery. The colostomy can be done electively before discharge from the nursery while the GI tract is decompressed by dilatation of the fistulous tract. A single orifice is diagnostic of a persistent cloacal defect usually accompany with a small-looking genitalia. Cloacas are associated to distended vaginas (hydrocolpos) and urologic malformations. This makes a sonogram of abdomen very important in the initial management of these babies for screening of obstructive uropathy (hydronephrosis and hydroureter).

Hydrocolpos can cause compressive obstruction of the bladder trigone and interfere with ureteral drainage. Failure to gain weight and frequents episodes of urinary tract infections shows a poorly drained urologic system. A colostomy in cloacas is indicated. 10% of babies will not pass meconium and will develop progressive abdominal distension. Radiological evaluation will be of help along with a diverting colostomy in this cases. Perineal fistulas can be managed with cutback without colostomy during the neonatal period.

Duplications

Duplications of the gastrointestinal tract are considered uncommon congenital anomalies usually diagnosed or unexpectedly encountered intraoperatively during the first two years of life. The duplicated bowelcan occur anywhere in the GI tract, is attached to the mesenteric border of the native bowel, shares a common wall and blood supply, coated with smooth muscle, and the epithelial lining is GI mucosa. May contain ectopic gastric or pancreatic tissue. Most are saccular, other tubular. Theories on their origin (split notochord syndrome, twining, faulty solid-stage recanalization) do not explain all cases of duplicated bowel. Three-fourth are found in the abdomen (most commonly the ileum and jejunum), 20% in the thorax, the rest thoraco-abdominal or cervical. Symptoms vary according to the size and location of the duplication. Clinical manifestations can range from intestinal obstruction, abdominal pain, GI bleeding, ulceration, or mediastinal compression. Ultrasound confirms the cystic nature of the lesion (muscular rim sign) and CT the relationship to surrounding structures. Management consist of surgical excision avoiding massive loss of normal bowel and removing all bowel suspect of harboring ectopic gastric mucosa.

Intussusception

Although intussusception can occur at any age, the greatest incidence occurs in infants between 4-10 months of age. Over half of the cases are in the first year of life. Frequently occurs after a recent upper respiratory infection, by Adenovirus type 3 that causes a reactive lymphoid hyperplasia that act as lead point (of Peyer's patch). A definite lead point is identified in about 5% of patients. These include: Meckel's diverticulum, polyps, Henoch's Schönlein purpura, hematoma, lymphoma, foreign bodies, and duplications. Most children have no lead point and it is felt that enlarged mesenteric nodes or swollen Peyer's patches may be the cause. The baby has intermittent periods of severe discomfort with screaming, stiffening and drawing up of the legs, followed by periods of rest. Vomiting may occur and bloody, mucoid (currant jelly) stool may be passed. The baby may become dehydrated and appear acutely ill. Frequently, lethargy may be an early sign. The diagnosis is made by barium enema, and hydrostatic reduction of the intussusception with barium is successful in approximately 50% of cases. To be successful, the barium must reflux into the terminal ileum. The surgeon should be notified before an attempt at barium reduction, and should be present at the time of study. Recently the use of gas enema reduction has been successful in patients with: (i) symptoms less than 12 hours, (ii) no rectal bleeding, (iii) absence of small bowel obstruction, and (iv) normally hydrated. Ultrasonography can be used as a rapid sensitive screening procedure in the initial diagnosis of intussusception.

Previous adverse clinical features that precluded barium reduction can be replaced during gas reduction. Predictors of failure of reduction are: (i) ileocolic intussusception, (ii) long duration of symptoms, (iii) rectal bleeding, and (iv) failed reduction at another institution. Air reduction (pneumocolon) is a very effective alternative method since it brings less radiation (shorter fluoroscopy time), less costs and less morbidity in cases of perforations. Failure of hydrostatic reduction requires urgent operation through a right lower quadrant horizontal incision.

The intussusception is reduced by pushing on the distal bowel like a tube of toothpaste rather than pulling the proximal bowel. Most cases are ileo-colic intussusception, and a few are jejuno-jejunal or ileo-ileal intussusception.

Appendicitis

Included in this group because is caused by obstruction of the appendiceal lumen, most commonly by fecaliths. When obstruction occurs, secretions from the appendix accumulates and acutely distends the lumen. The pressure eventually produces arterial obstruction leading to infarction. Bacteria initially invade the mucosa and produce intramural infection. Other causes include pinworm infestation, carcinoids and lymphoid hyperplasia. Initially periumbilical pain secondary to distension of the lumen of the appendix occurs. Pain impulses from the wall of the distended appendix are carried by visceral afferent sympathetic fibers through the celiac ganglion to T10 and then referred to the umbilical area in the tenth dermatome. Later the pain shifts to the right lower quadrant of the abdomen, where it localizes. The shift in location is an important diagnostic sign and indicates the formation of irritating exudate around the inflamed appendix that stimulates the pain receptors of the peritoneum locally. Anorexia, nausea and vomiting follow the onset of abdominal pain. Physical findings include an obviously ill-appearing child who usually will walk slowly and bent over. Motion, heel tap, or bouncing on the heels will elicit pain in the right lower quadrant. Point tenderness in the right lower quadrant (or the persistence of right lower quadrant pain) is the most reliable physical finding. There is usually rebound and referred pain to the right lower quadrant, indicating peritoneal inflammation. Fever is usually present. Laboratory findings are an elevated white blood cell count in most instances. Very high WBC's > 18,000 may indicate perforation. Urinalyses is generally clear, but occasionally RBC's or WBC's may be associated with the inflamed appendix adjacent to the bladder or ureter. Radiographic findings may include ileus, appendicolith (pathognomonic finding), splinting, abdominal wall edema, and only very rarely, free air. Initial treatment is rehydration to establish adequate urinary output. Any evidence of possible perforation should mandate the use of appropriate antibiotics. Once adequate then surgical intervention proceeds quickly. Most patients are approached through a right lower quadrant horizontal muscle splitting incision. Removal of the appendix, irrigation and, when localized abscesses are identified, institution of drainage. Appendicitis is usually diagnosed from signs, symptoms, results of simple laboratory tests a/o simple abdominal films. After simple abdominal films an appendicolith (coprolith, fecalith, retained barium or foreign body) is sometimes found in the symptomatic child with right lower quadrant pain or less commonly in an asymptomatic situation. In the child WITH SYMPTOMS of low abdominal pain this finding should be followed by appendectomy. Appendiceal fecaliths and calculi play a role in the pathogenesis of appendicitis and are associated with perforation and gangrene. In the ASYMPTOMATIC situation a prophylactic appendectomy is NOT justified when an appendicolith, retained barium or another foreign body within the lumen of the appendix is identified. A normal appendix will expel the appendicolith or barium in a variable period. The parents should be informed that appendicitis may develop and that the child should seek a physician if abdominal symptoms develop. A note should appear in the record explaining this conversation. A word on incidental appendectomy: Removing a normal appendix incidentally during a surgical procedure done for reasons other than abdominal pain is associated with a small but definite increase in adverse postoperative outcome. In this respect incidental appendectomy has been found to increase the incidence of postoperative septic complications (wound infection). Incidental appendectomy is indicated in procedures where a potential diagnostic pitfall can occur such as Ladd procedure for malrotation, diagnostic laparoscopy for right quadrant pain and surgically reduced ileo-colic intussusception.

Chronic Intestinal Pseudo-Obstruction

Chronic Intestinal Pseudo-Obstruction is a rare disorder of intestinal motility in infants and children characterized by recurrent attacks of abdominal pain, distension, vomiting, constipation and weight loss in the absence of obvious mechanical lesions. The disease can be familial or sporadic. Suggested etiology is degeneration of enteric nervous or smooth muscle cells. The diagnosis is based on history, physical exam, radiographies and motility studies. X-Ray hallmarks are: absent strictures, absent, decreased or disorganized intestinal motility, and dilated small/large bowel loops. Associated conditions identified in 10-30% of patients are bladder dysfunction (megacystis) and neurological problems. Histologic pattern portrayed: myenteric plexus hyperplasia, glial cell hyperplasia, and small ganglion cells (hypoganglionosis). Management is primary supportive: intestinal decompression (NG), long-term TPN and antibiotic prophylaxis. Motility agents are unsuccessful. Venting gastrostomy with home parenteral nutrition has shortened the high hospitalization rate associated to this disease process. A similar condition can be seen in early fed prematures due to immaturity of intestinal motility.

Meconium-related Disease

1. *Meconium Ileus:* Meconium Ileus (MI) is a neonatal intraluminal intestinal obstruction associated with Cystic Fibrosis(10-20%). The distal ileum is packed with an abnormally thick, viscous, inspissated meconium. The meconium has a reduced water

content the result of decreased pancreatic enzyme activity and a prolonged small bowel intestinal transit time. MI can be classified as simple or complicated. Simple MI appears in the first 48 hrs of life with abdominal distension and bilious vomiting. Complicated MI is more severe (< 24 hrs) with progressive abdominal distension, respiratory distress, and peritonitis. X-Ray findings are: dilated bowel loops, absent air-fluid levels, "soap-bubble" granular appearance of distal ileum due to a mixture of air with the tenacious meconium. Therapy consists of Gastrografin enema for simple cases: hyperosmolar solution draws fluid to the bowel lumen causing an osmotic diarrhea. Operative therapy is reserved for failed gastrografin attempts and complicated cases (associated to volvulus, atresias, gangrene, perforation or peritonitis). Surgical procedures has included: ileostomy with irrigation, resection with anastomosis, and resection with ileostomy (Mikulicz and Bishop-Kopp). Post-operative management includes: 10% acetylcysteine p.o., oral feedings (pregestimil), pancreatic enzyme replacement, and prophylactic pulmonary therapy. Long-term prognosis depends on the degree of severity and progression of cystic fibrosis pulmonary disease.

2. *Meconium Peritonitis:* Meconium peritonitis (MP) is a chemical peritonitis that occurs following bowel perforation during fetal life. It is generally looked upon as benign, resulting in no long-term sequelae. The peritonitis occurs when the meconium leaves the bowel, enters the peritoneal cavity and spreads throughout causing a sterile inflammatory reaction. Most common site of bowel perforation is the distal ileum, and 50% of babies with MP develop intestinal obstruction. Prenatal ultrasound findings include ascites, intraabdominal masses, bowel dilatation and the development of intraabdominal calcifications. Bowel disorders which lead to MP in utero are those resulting in bowel obstruction

and perforation, such as small bowel atresias, volvulus and meconium ileus. MP can be divided into simple or complex. Cases with spontaneously healed perforation (simple MP) need observation as they rarely develop symptoms. Newborns with complex MP are born with bowel obstruction a/or pseudocyst formation (localized collection of meconium contained in a cyst made of fibrous granulation tissue). Complex MP needs surgical therapy.

3. *Meconium plug syndrome/Left hypoplastic colon syndrome:* Colonic obstruction in the newborn child could be the result of necrotizing enterocolitis, atresia, meconium plug syndrome, duplication cyst, Hirschsprung disease or the small left colon syndrome. In meconium plug syndrome the baby expels a grey-meconium and the obstruction subsides. Meconium plug syndrome (MPS) was first described by Clatworthy in 1956 as a transient form of distal colonic or rectal obstruction in newborns caused by an inspissated, immobile meconium. The plug is white and chalky and rarely involves the small bowel. Clinical manifestations include progressive abdominal distension, vomiting (sometimes is bilious) and failure to pass meconium during the initial two days of life. Though most cases are idiopathic, MPS has been associated with prematurity, hypotonia, hypermagnesemia (reduces acetylcholine release with subsequent myoneural depression), diabetic mother, Hirschsprung's disease and cystic fibrosis. Colonic contrast study suggests the diagnosis (filling defect) and can be therapeutic in most cases to relieve the obstruction. Gastrografin instillation is highly effective in moving the obstructing long, thick plug, even in tiny premature infants with MPS. Suction rectal biopsy to exclude the diagnosis of Hirschsprung's disease along with cystic fibrosis screening is warranted in all cases of MPS. The diagnosis of MPS is made after all the above causes are

excluded. Need for surgery is extremely rare. The left (small) hypoplastic colon syndrome (LHCS) is a very rare cause of colonic obstruction identified in newborns with characteristic roentgenographic features resembling those of Hirschsprung's disease. Manifesting in the first 24-48 hours of life, LHCS is a functional disturbance related to immaturity of the intrinsic innervation of the colon that is especially common in low birth weight neonates or of diabetic mothers. Intestinal perforation, sepsis, hypoglycemia and death may occur. The diagnosis is suggested in a barium enema when the caliber of the left colon is small with a transitional zone at the splenic flexure. Management consists of hypoglycemia correction, antibiotics, nasogastric decompression and observation. In most babies the obstruction clears in 48-72 hours. When the clinical diagnosis is not readily apparent a rectal biopsy and sweat chloride test should be done to differentiate LHCS from Hirschsprung disease and cystic fibrosis respectively. The narrowed left colon remains narrow in follow-up.

HERNIAS, THORACIC CONDITIONS AND ABDOMINAL WALL DEFECTS

Diaphragmatic Hernia

Congenital Diaphragmatic Hernia (Bochdalek)

The most common congenital diaphragmatic hernia (CDH) is that which occurs through the posterolateral defect of Bochdalek. It is caused by failure of the pleuroperitoneal membrane to develop adequately and close before the intestines returning to the abdomen at the tenth week of gestation. The intestines then enter the pleural cavity and cause poor lung development leading to pulmonary hypoplasia (a reduced number of alveoli per area of lung tissue). This defect is postero-lateral in the diaphragm and may vary in size. Stomach, liver or spleen may be partly in chest as well. Frequency is 1:2000 live births and the natural history in prenatally diagnosed CDH is that 60% will die. The clinical presentation is that the newborn becomes rapidly cyanotic, acidotic, and has poor ventilation. Major findings relate to the degree of pulmonary maldevelopment. Chest films will show intestines in the chest. Left sided hernias are more common than right (90% on left). Placement of a radiopaque nasogastric tube may show the tube coiled in the lower left chest. Higher risk factors are: early appearance of symptoms in life, prematurity and associated anomalies. Treatment consist of rapid intubation and ventilation with use of muscle relaxants, placement of a nasogastric tube to prevent gaseous distension of the intestines and preoperative stabilization of arterial blood gases and acid-base status. Surgery can be undertaken when one of the following objectives are met:

1. Blood gases normalize with no significant changes between preductal and postductal samples,
2. Echocardiogram demonstrate reduce pulmonary pressure and pulmonary peripheral resistance.

Operative management consist of abdominal approach, closure of hernia by primary repair or use of mesh, and correction of malrotation. Postoperative management is very difficult. Due to hypoplastic lungs, there is frequently pulmonary hypertension leading to right-to-left shunting and progressive hypoxemia, hypercarbia, and acidosis that worsens the pulmonary hypertension. The use of chest tubes may cause overstretching of the already hypoplastic alveoli causing: increase pulmonary hypertension, reduce functional residual capacity and reduce lung compliance. Postoperatively, the infant should be kept paralyzed and ventilated and only very slowly weaned from the ventilator. The severity of pulmonary hypoplasia, both ipsilaterally and contralaterally, is the main determinant of outcome. ECMO (extracorporeal membrane oxygenator) has come to reduce somewhat the mortality of this condition.

The mortality of CDH is directly related to the degree of lung hypoplasia associated. Death is caused by persistent pulmonary hypertension and right ventricular failure. Prospective studies of prenatally diagnosed fetus prior to 25 wk. gestation has shown that 60% will die despite optimal postnatal care. This unsolved problem has prompted investigators to develop new treatment options such as preoperative stabilization, jetfrequency ventilation, and ECMO. Another area of development is intrauterine fetal surgical repair. To achieve success fetal surgery should:

1. Pose no risk to the mother (innocent bystander) or her future reproductive capacity;
2. Tocolytic therapy in the post-op weeks should proved effective to avoid prenatal stillbirths; and
3. The procedure should be superior to conventional therapy. Intrauterine repair has meet with limited success due to herniation of the fetal liver into the chest through the defect. Disturbance of the umbilical circulation during or after liver reduction causes fetal death. Positive-pressure ventilation after birth reduces the liver before the baby comes for surgical repair. the left lateral segment of the liver. Another less invasive approach is enlarging the hypoplastic lungs by reducing the normal egress of fetal lung fluid with controlled tracheal obstruction called PLUGS (Plug Lung Until it Grows). Delayed presentation beyond the neonatal period is rare, estimated to occur in 4-6% of cases. Infants and children will present with either respiratory or gastrointestinal symptoms such as: chronic respiratory tract infection, vomiting, intermittent intestinal obstruction, and feeding difficulty. Occasionally the child is asymptomatic. The small size of the defect protected by either the spleen or the liver and the presence of a hernial sac may delay the intestinal herniation into the chest. A rise intraabdominal pressure by coughing or vomiting transmitted to any defect of the diaphragm

makes visceral herniation more likely. Diagnosis is confirmed by chest or gastrointestinal contrast imaging. Management consists of immediate surgery after preop stabilization. Most defects can be closed primarily through an abdominal approach. Chest-tube placement in the non-hypoplastic lung is of help. Surgical results are generally excellent. A few deaths have resulted from cardiovascular and respiratory compromise due to visceral herniation causing mediastinal and pulmonary compression.

Morgagni Hernias

Morgagni Hernias (MH) are rare congenital diaphragmatic defects close to the anterior midline between the costal and sternal origin of the diaphragm. They occur retrosternally in the midline or more commonly on either side (parasternally) of the junction of the embryologic septum transversum and thoracic wall representing less than 2% of all diaphragmatic defects. Almost always asymptomatic, typically present in older children or adults with minimal gastrointestinal symptoms or as incidental finding during routine chest radiography (mass or air-fluid levels). Infants may develop respiratory symptoms (tachypnea, dyspnea and cyanosis) with distress. Cardiac tamponade due to protrusion into the pericardial cavity has been reported. The MH defect contains a sac with liver, small/ large bowel as content. Associated conditions are: heart defects, trisomy 21, omphalocele, and Cantrell' pentalogy. US and CT-Scan can demonstrate the defect. Management is operative. Transabdominal subcostal approach is preferred with reduction of the defect and suturing of the diaphragm to undersurface of sternum and posterior rectus sheath. Large defects with phrenic nerve displacement may need a thoracic approach. Results after surgery rely on associated conditions.

Hiatal Hernia

Hiatal hernia is rarely a problem in infants unless associated with gastroesophageal reflux or severe anatomic dysfunction of the stomach (upside-down intrathoracic stomach). Two types of esophageal hernia recognized are the hiatal and paraesophageal hernia. Diagnosis is made radiologically always and in a number of patients endoscopically. The hiatal hernia (HH) refers to herniation of the stomach to the chest through the esophageal hiatus. The lower esophageal sphincter also moves. It can consist of a small transitory epiphrenic loculation (minor) up to an upside-down intrathoracic stomach (major). HH generally develops due to a congenital, traumatic or iatrogenic factor. Most disappear by the age of two years, but all forms of HH can lead to peptic esophagitis from Gastroesophageal reflux. Repair of HH is determined by the pathology of its associated reflux (causing failure to thrive, esophagitis, stricture, respiratory symptoms) or the presence of the stomach in the thoracic cavity. In the paraesophageal hernia (PH) variety the stomach migrates to the chest and the lower esophageal sphincter stays in its normal anatomic position. PH is a frequent problem after antireflux operations in patients without posterior crural repair. Small PH can be observed. With an increase in size or appearance of symptoms (reflux, gastric obstruction, bleeding, infarction or perforation) the PH should be repaired. The incidence of PH has increased with the advent of the laparoscopic fundoplication.

Lung Bud Anomalies

Congenital Lobar Emphysema

Congenital lobar emphysema (CLE) is an unusual lung bud anomaly characterized by massive air trapping in the lung parenchyma that nearly always occurs in infancy and affects males more commonly (2:1). Lobar over distension causes compression of adjacent lung tissue, mediastinal shift and decrease in venous return. When this occurs persistent progressive respiratory distress (dyspnea, tachypnea, wheezing, cough and cyanosis) develops requiring lobectomy. Asymptomatic CLE exists, more commonly beyond infancy and associated with an acute viral respiratory infection. Lobar hyperinflation, flat diaphragms and retrosternal air, mediastinal shift in simple films suggests the diagnosis. CT scan depicts the abnormal anatomy (lung herniation) and the morphology of the remaining lung. V/Q scans confirm the non-functioning nature of the affected lobe. Upper and middle right lobes are more commonly affected. Etiology centers in a combination of bronchial (flap/valve) obstruction with congenital cartilage dysplasia. Most common associated defect is cardiovascular (VSD, PDA). Symptomatic patients nearly always require lobectomy. Asymptomatic children do not benefit from surgical treatment but need close follow-up. Prenatally diagnosed cases need referral to surgery centers.

Pulmonary Sequestration

Pulmonary sequestrations refer to masses of abnormal lung parenchyma with anomalous systemic blood supply not communicating with the normal tracheobronchial tree. The abnormal lung parenchyma may be Intralobar (IS) or Extralobar Sequestration (ES). Intralobar is contained within the visceral pleural of a lower lobe receiving the blood supply from the abdominal aorta or other thoracic vessel. It is believed IS are acquired postinfectious process due to their association with chronic recurrent lung infection and reactive airway disease. ES is a congenital malformation with variable ectopic blood supply (aorta) having its own pleural investment separate from normal lung, containing typical features of CCAM-2 (40%) and associated malformations (40%). Both types can have patent communication with foregut. Prenatal diagnosis can be obtained with real-time US with Doppler imaging (can cause fetal lung compression, mediastinal shifts and hydrops). Postnatally, contrast-enhanced CT may establish the diagnosis eliminating the need for more invasive imaging (arteriography). Most presents in early infancy with a soft tissue opacity in the posterior basal segments of the lung on simple chest films. Management consists of resection to alleviate symptoms and avoid complications. ES can be managed with resection alone, while IS needs lobectomy. Anecdotal cases of partial or total disappearance of these masses while asymptomatic has been reported.

Cystic Adenomatoid Malformation

Congenital cystic adenomatoid malformation is a lung bud lesion characterize by dysplasia of respiratory epithelium caused by overgrowth of distal bronchiolar tissue. Prenatally diagnosed CCAM prognosis depends on the size of the lung lesion and can cause: mediastinal shift, hypoplasia of normal lung tissue, polyhydramnios, and fetal hydrops (cardiovascular shunt). Classified in two types based on ultrasound findings: macrocystic (lobar, > 5 mm cysts, anechoic, favorable prognosis) and microcystic (diffuse, more solid, echogenic, lethal). Occurs as an isolated (sporadic) event with a low rate of recurrence. Survival depends on histology. Hydrops is caused by vena caval obstruction, heart compression and mediastinal shift. The natural history is that some will decrease in size, while others disappear. Should be follow with serial sonograms. Prenatal management for impending fetal hydrops has consisted of thoraco-amniotic shunts (dislodge, migrate and occlude), and intra-uterine fetal resection (technically feasible, reverses hydrops, allows lung growth). Postnatal management consist of lobectomy.

Bronchogenic Cyst

Bronchogenic cysts (BC), first described in 1911, are benign congenital lesions of the respiratory tract that have the potential to develop complications creating a dilemma in diagnosis and treatment. BC are commonly located in the mediastinum (2/3) or lung parenchyma (1/3) arising from anomalous budding along the primitive tracheobronchial tube (foregut duplication errors). Other atypical locations are cervical, subcutaneous, paravertebral, etc. Contain mucoid material lined with ciliated columnar epithelium (bronchial glands, smooth muscle, cartilage) not communicating with the respiratory tract. Clinical presentation may range from prenatal diagnosis, asymptomatic (1/3) lesions identified during routine work-up to symptomatic (2/3) cases. Infants may show respiratory distress: cough, dyspnea, cyanosis, hemoptysis or dysphagia. Older children present with chest pain, non-productive cough or pulmonary infection. Diagnosis relies on chest films and CT-Scan. Bronchoscopy and barium swallow are not very useful. Infection, hemorrhage, erosion, malignant potential and expansion mandate surgical management consisting of thoracotomy with excision of the lesion if mediastinal in location, and segmentectomy or lobectomy for intraparenchymal cysts. Marsupialization is associated with recurrence.

Inguinal Hernias, Hydroceles, Undescended Testis and Epigastric Hernias

A hernia is defined as a protrusion of a portion of an organ or tissue through an abnormal opening. For groin (inguinal or femoral) hernias, this protrusion is into a hernial sac. Whether or not the mere presence of a hernial sac (or processus vaginalis) constitutes a hernia is debated. Inguinal hernias in children are almost exclusively indirect type. Those rare instances of direct inguinal hernia are caused by previous surgery and floor disruption. An indirect inguinal hernia protrudes through the internal inguinal ring, within the cremaster fascia, extending down the spermatic cord for varying distances. The direct hernia protrudes through the posterior wall of the inguinal canal, i.e., medial to deep inferior epigastric vessels, destroying or stretching the transversalis fascia. The embryology of indirect inguinal hernia is as follows: the duct descending to the testicle is a small offshoot of the great peritoneal sac in the lower abdomen. During the third month of gestation, the processus vaginalis extends down toward the scrotum and follows the chorda gubernaculum that extends from the testicle or the retroperitoneum to the scrotum. During the seventh month, the testicle descend into the scrotum, where the processus vaginalis forms a covering for the testicle and the serous sac in which it resides. At about the time of birth, the portion of the processus vaginalis between the testicle and the abdominal cavity obliterates, leaving a peritoneal cavity separate from the tunica vaginalis that surrounds the testicle. Approximately 1-3% of children have a hernia. For infants born prematurely, the incidence varies from 3-5%. The typical patient with an inguinal hernia has an intermittent lump or bulge in the groin, scrotum, or labia noted at times of increased intra-abdominal pressure. A communicating hydrocele is always associated with a hernia. This hydrocele fluctuates in size and is usually larger in ambulatory patients at the end of the day. If a loop of bowel becomes entrapped (incarcerated) in a hernia, the patient develops pain followed by signs of intestinal obstruction. If not reduced, compromised blood supply (strangulation) leads to perforation and peritonitis. Most incarcerated hernias in children can be reduced. The incidence of inguinal hernia (IH) in premature babies (9-11%) is higher than full-term (3-5%), with a dramatic risk of incarceration (30%). Associated to these episodes of incarceration are chances of: gonadal infarction (the undescended testes complicated by a hernia are more vulnerable to vascular compromise and atrophy), bowel obstruction and strangulation. Symptomatic hernia can complicate the clinical course of babies at NICU ill with hyaline membrane, sepsis, NEC and other conditions needing ventilatory support. Repair should be undertaken before hospital discharge to avoid complications. Prematures have: poorly developed respiratory control center, collapsible rib cage, deficient fatigue-resistant muscular fibers in the diaphragm that predispose then to potential life-threatening post-op respiratory complications such as: need of assisted ventilation (most common), apnea and bradycardia, emesis, cyanosis and re-intubation (due to laryngospasm). Independent risk factors associated to this complications are:

1. History of RDS/bronchopulmonary dysplasia,
2. History of patent ductus arteriosus,
3. Low absolute weight (< 1.5 Kg), and
4. Anemia (Hgb < 10 gm- is associated to a higher incidence of post-op apnea). Postconceptual age (sum of intra- and extrauterine life) has been cited as the factor having greatest impact on post-op complications.

These observation makes imperative that preemies (with post conceptual age of less than 45 weeks) be carefully monitored in-hospital for at least 24 hours after surgical repair of their hernias. Outpatient repair is safer for those prematures above the 60 wk. Of postconceptual age. The very low birth weight infant with symptomatic hernia can benefit from epidural anesthesia. At times, the indirect inguinal hernia will extend into the scrotum and can be reduced by external, gentle pressure. Occasionally, the hernia will present as a bulge in the soft tissue overlying the internal ring. It is sometimes difficult to demonstrate and the physician must rely on the patient's history of an intermittent bulge in the groin seen with crying, coughing or straining. Elective herniorrhaphy at a near convenient time is treatment of choice. Since risk of incarceration is high in children, repair should be undertaken shortly after diagnosis. Simple high ligation of the sac is all that is required. Pediatric patients are allowed to return to full activity immediately after hernia repair. Patients presenting with incarceration should have an attempt at reduction (possible in greater than 98% with experience), and then admission for repair during that hospitalization. Bilateral exploration is done routinely by most experienced pediatric surgeons. Recently the use of groin laparoscopy through the hernial sac permits visualization of the contralateral side. Approximately 1% of females with inguinal hernias will have the testicular feminization syndrome.

A hydrocele is a collection of fluid in the space surrounding the testicle between the layers of the tunica vaginalis. Hydroceles can be scrotal, of the cord, abdominal, or a combination of the above. A hydrocele of the cord is the fluid-filled remnant of the processus vaginalis separated from the tunica vaginalis. A communicating hydrocele is one that communicates with the peritoneal cavity by way of a narrow opening into a hernial sac. Hydroceles are common in infants. Some are associated with an inguinal hernia. They are often bilateral, and like hernias, are more common on the right than the left. Most hydroceles will resolved spontaneously by 1-2 years of age. After this time, elective repair can be performed at any time. Operation is done through the groin and search made for an associated hernia. Aspiration of a hydrocele should never be attempted. As a therapeutic measure it is ineffective, and as a diagnostic tool it is a catastrophe if a loop of bowel is entrapped. A possible exception to this is the postoperative recurrent hydrocele. The ndescended testis is a term we use to describe all instances in which the testis cannot be manually manipulated into the scrotum. The testes form from the medial portion of the urogenital ridge extending from the diaphragm into the pelvis. In arrested descent, they may be found from the kidneys to the internal inguinal ring. Rapid descent through the internal inguinal ring commences at approximately week 28, the left testis preceding the right. Adequate amounts of male hormones are necessary for descent.The highest levels of male hormones in the maternal circulation have been demonstrated at week 28. Thus, it appears that failure of descent may be related to inadequate male hormone levels or to failure of the end-organ to respond.The undescended testes may be found from the hilum of the kidney to the external inguinal ring. A patent processus vaginalis or true hernial sac will be present 90% of the time. The incidence is about 0.28% of the population, approximately 50% occurs on the right, 25% on the left, and 25% occur bilaterally. The diagnosis of undescended testes is usually made by the parents or first examining physician. The important point is the absolute necessity of distinguishing between retractile testes and the true undescended testes. Testes that can be drawn to the scrotum, even if they retract again, are retractile testes and not undescended, the squatting position may aid in helping descend the testes for exam. Retractile testis need no further surgical management.

Since Leydig cell degeneration can occur after age two, present recommendations are for orchiopexy before age 2. Although testicular malignancy is rare, undescended testes have a 40-50 times higher incidence of developing seminomas. This can occur in the contralateral normally descended testis as well as the undescended testis. Surgical repair does not reduce the incidence of malignancy, but does allow for examination and earlier detection. Another reason for surgical repair is the higher incidence of trauma and torsion in the undescended testis. Bilateral undescended testes may be initially treated with a four-week course of human chorionic gonadotrophin. Approximately 15-30% of patients will have descent with this therapy. Surgical repair is most commonly performed by a Dartos pouch technique. Laparoscopy helps in non-palpable undescended testis by identifying those testis that did not developed, suffered an ischemic intrauterine event, and in performing first stage Steven-Fowler technique.

Congenital epigastric defects occur anywhere in the linea alba from the navel to the xiphoid process.

They represent almost 5% of all hernias defect that presents in children. Most epigastric hernias occur in the midline, are small (15-25 mm), asymptomatic and reducible. Multiple fascial defects can also be present in 20% of all cases. The defect might arise congenitally from an abnormally wide orifice of a blood vessel during development of the linea alba. The bump is the result of a piece of preperitoneal fat stuck through the fascial defect. Tenderness is an unusual symptom while growth of the defect occurs with time. Most surgeons recommend repair of the defect at the time of presentation. Repair is an outpatient procedure done under general anesthesia with low morbidity and risk of recurrence. Voluminous epigastric hernia (5-10 cm) with a sac that contains epiploic appendages or viscera (ileum loops, stomach) has also been rarely reported in infants.

Mediastinal Cysts

Mediastinal cysts identified in children are classified according to the compartment where they arise as: anterior (extends to the sternum, thoracic inlet and anterior border of the heart), middle (between anterior mediastinum and anterior borders of the vertebrae) or posterior mediastinum. Although usually asymptomatic, they require excision for purpose of diagnosis and avoidance of symptoms such as chest pain, airway obstruction, hemoptysis or dysphagia. Diagnosis can be accomplished with the use of CT-Scan, US and esophagogram. Some of the most common encounter cysts in the mediastinum are: bronchogenic cysts, neurenteric cysts, pericardial cysts, cystic hygroma, thymic and dermoid cysts.

Umbilical Hernias

Between the sixth and tenth gestational week, the developing gastrointestinal tract is partially extruded into the umbilical cord with return into the abdomen by the tenth week. By the time of birth, the umbilical ring has become entirely closed by the developing abdominal wall except for the space occupied by the cord, which contains the umbilical vein, paired umbilical arteries, and the fibrous remnants of the urachus and omphalomesenteric duct (yolk sac). After ligation of the cord, the vessels thrombosed and the cord dries and sloughs off, leaving a granulating surface that heals by cicatrization and is covered by epithelium. This is followed by scar contraction and retraction of the umbilicus. It is believed that most umbilical hernias occur through the cephalad portion of the umbilical ring, where the contracted scar around the obliterated umbilical vein is less dense than in the caudal portion of the scar. Umbilical hernias are very common, especially in prematures, blacks, and certain syndromes, such as Down's. The incidence decrease with age since many will close spontaneously. The diagnosis is made by physical exam, there is a fascial defect at the umbilicus.Complications such as strangulation or incarceration are extremely rare in children.**Umbilical strapping should not be done** since it does not promotes closure and may lead to skin erosion. Elective repair is usually delayed until after five years of age since closure may occur spontaneously or the defect may get smaller, allowing easier repair. Operative repair includes excision of the sac and horizontal one-layer closure through a small infraumbilical incision.

Omphalocele and Gastroschisis

The three most common abdominal wall defect in newborns are umbilical hernia, gastroschisis and omphalocele. Referral to tertiary centers with available neonatal intensive care is necessary in prenatally diagnosed cases. Changing the route of delivery does not affect outcome for either defect. Omphalocele has a high incidence of associated anomalies (cardiac, neurogenic, genitourinary, skeletal, chromosomal syndromes) that are the cornerstones of mortality. Detailed search for associated anomalies, fetal echocardiogram and karyotyping should be performed always. Cesarean section is justified in large omphaloceles (> 5 cm) to avoid liver damage, sac rupture and dystocia. Gastroschisis prenatal US appearance depends on gestational age and condition of extruded bowel. Fetal karyotyping testing is less important.Intestinal atresia complicates the defect, the result of an intrauterine vascular accident. Intestinal obstruction due to atresia or luminal constriction may cause polyhydramnios, fetal growth retardation and preterm labor, findings that can be monitored with serial US. No benefit has been found in recommending routine c-section for most cases of gastroschisis. Preterm deliveries by c-section have been found to prevent bowel damage in fetus with progressive bowel dilatation and thickening, a finding that has not been corroborated by others. Abnormal US appearance of fetal bowel is associated with more bowel edema, longer operative time and a higher incidence of postoperative complications. Omphalocele is a milder form of primary abdominoschisis since during the embryonic folding process the outgrowth at the umbilical ring is insufficient (shortage in apoptotic cell death). Bowel and/or viscera remains in the umbilical cord causing a large abdominal wall defect. Defect may have liver, spleen, stomach, and bowel in the sac while the abdominal cavity remains underdeveloped in size. The sac is composed of chorium, Wharton's jelly and peritoneum. The defect is centrally localized and measures 4-10 cm in diameter. A small defect of less than 2 cm with bowel inside is referred as a hernia of the umbilical cord. There is a high incidence (30-60%)of associated anomalies in patients with omphalocele. Epigastric localized omphalocele are associated with sternal and intracardiac defects (i.e., **Pentalogy of Cantrell**), and hypogastric omphalocele have a high association with genito-urinary defects (i.e., Cloacal Exstrophy). All have malrotation. Cardiac, neurogenic, genitourinary, skeletal and chromosomal changes and syndromes are the cornerstones of mortality. Antenatal diagnosis may affect management by stimulating search for associated anomalies and changing the site, mode or timing of delivery. Cesarean section is warranted in large omphaloceles to avoid liver damage and dystocia. After initial stabilization management requires consideration of the size of defect, prematurity and associated anomalies. Primary closure with correction of the malrotation should be attempted whenever possible. If this is not possible, then a plastic mesh/ silastic chimney is fashioned around the defect to cover the intestinal contents and the contents slowly reduced over 5-14 days. Antibiotics and nutritional support are mandatory. Manage control centers around sepsis, respiratory status, liver and bowel dysfunction from increased intraabdominal pressure. The exact embryology of gastroschisis is unclear. The defect is always to the right of the midline with a normally attached umbilical cord. Theories include failure of the right lateral somatopleure to form properly, intrauterine rupture and intrauterine vascular accident leading to ischemia of the right developing rectus. Associated anomalies are rare, with an 11% incidence of atresia. Treatment is identical to omphalocele except more urgent to avoid problems with the exposed bowel (dehydration and hypothermia). More than 90% babies survived. Prenatal diagnosis has brought a controversy toward optimal mode of delivery (Cesarean vs vaginal). The appearance of the bowel is edematous, matted and foreshortened due to exposure to amniotic fluid, and the constrictive vascular effects of a small defect.

Femoral Hernias

Femoral hernias (FH) in the pediatric age are very rare accounting for less than 0.5% of all groin hernias in children. Children present with a recurrent groin lump that is usually reducible. The correct preoperative diagnosis is often overlooked. FH is defined as a protrusion of viscera, fat or omentum occurring through the femoral hiatus. Peak incidence occurs between five and ten years of age. Misdiagnoses include inguinal hernia, lymphadenitis, and lymphangioma. Preoperative diagnosis is possible if the bulge appears in a location inferior and lateral to that of the commonly occurring indirect hernia. Early recurrence of a groin swelling after what seems to be an adequate inguinal herniorrhaphy should be suspected of having a missed femoral hernia. Mc Vay expressed that the etiology was a congenitally narrow posterior inguinal wall attachment into Cooper's ligament with a resultant enlarged femoral ring. Excision of the sac and repair of the femoral canal is curative. At surgery Cooper's ligament (Mc Vay) repair is the surgical treatment of choice, though some contend that simple repair of the femoral ring carries good long-term results.

GASTROINTESTINAL BLEEDING

Upper GI bleeding (Neonate)

Initially do an Apt test to determine if blood comes from fetal origin or maternal origin (blood swallowed by the fetus). If its of fetal origin then consider a coagulation profile (PT, PTT). If this coagulation profile is normal the possibilities are either stress gastritis or ulcer disease. If the coagulation profile is abnormal then consider hematologic disease of the newborn and manage with vitamin K. The apt test is performed by mixing 1 part of vomitus with 5 part H2O, centrifuge the mixture and remove 5 ml (pink). Then add 1 ml 1% NaOH, wait 2 minutes and if it remains pinks is fetal blood, if it turns brown-yellow its maternal blood.

Lower GI bleeding (Neonate)

Again start with an Apt test, if its positive its maternal swallow blood, if its negative do a PT, PTT. If the coagulation profile is abnormal give Vit K for hematologic disorder of newborn. If it's normal do a rectal exam. A fissure could be the cause, if negative then consider either malrotation or Necrotizing enterocolitis.

Necrotizing Enterocolitis (NEC)

Although the exact pathogenesis of NEC is not known, the most widely held theory is that of perinatal stress leading to selective circulatory ischemia. The stress includes prematurity, sepsis, hypoxia, hypothermia, and jaundice. These babies frequently have umbilical artery, vein catheters, have received exchange transfusions or early feeds with hyperosmolar formulas. The intestinal mucosal cells are highly sensitive to ischemia and mucosal damage leads to bacterial invasion of the intestinal wall. Gas-forming organisms produce pneumatosis intestinalis (air in the bowel wall readily seen on abdominal films). Full-thickness necrosis leads to perforation, free air and abscess formation. These usually premature infants develop increased gastric residuals, abdominal distension, bloody stools, acidosis and dropping platelet count. The abdominal wall becomes reddened and edematous. There may be persistent masses and signs of peritonitis. Perforation leads to further hypoxia, acidosis and temperature instability. The acid-base status is monitored for worsening acidosis and hypoxia. Serial platelet counts are obtained and, with increasing sepsis, the platelet count drops <50,000, indicating intravascular coagulation and decreased bone marrow production. The white blood cell count may be high, low or normal and is not generally of help. Serial abdominal films are obtained to look for evidence of free abdominal air, a worsening picture of pneumatosis intestinalis, or free portal air. Therapy consist initially of stopping feeds, instituting nasogastric suctioning and beginning broad-spectrum antibiotics (ampicillin and gentamycin). Persistent or worsening clinical condition and sepsis or free air on abdominal films require urgent surgical intervention.

Attempts to preserve as much viable bowel as possible are mandatory to prevent resultant short gut syndrome.

Complicated NEC is the most common neonatal surgical emergency of modern times, has diverse etiologies, significant mortality and affects mostly premature babies. The use of primary peritoneal drain (PPD) in the management of NEC dates from 1977. The technique is used in the very low birth weight premature infant (<1500 gm) with pneumoperitoneum, metabolic and hemodynamic instability. Consist of a right lower quadrant incision and placement of a drainage (Penrose or catheter) under local anesthesia with subsequent irrigation performed bedside at the NICU. Initially used as a temporizing measure before formal laparotomy, some patient went to improvement without the need for further surgery (almost one-third). They either had an immature (fetal type) healing process or a focal perforation (not associated to NEC?) which healed spontaneously. Those babies not improved by PPD either die (20%), go on to laparotomy and half die (20%) or develop complications (24%). Some suggestion made are: PPD should be an adjunct to preop stabilization, before placing drain be sure pt has NEC by X-rays, persistent metabolic acidosis means uncontrolled peritoneal sepsis, do not place drain in pts with inflammatory mass or rapid development of intraperitoneal fluid, the longer the drainage the higher the need for laparotomy.

Upper GI Bleeding (Older Children)

In the initial evaluation a history should be obtained for bleeding disorders, skin lesions, and aspirin or steroid ingestion. The physical exam for presence of enlarged liver, spleen, masses, ascites, or evidence of trauma or portal hypertension. Labs such as bleeding studies and endoscopy, contrast studies if bleeding stops.

Common causes of Upper GI bleeding are:

1. Esophagus
   a. Varices- usually presents as severe upper gastrointestinal bleeding in a 2-3 year old who has previously been healthy except for problems in the neonatal period. This is a result of extra-hepatic portal obstruction (portal vein thrombosis most commonly), with resulting varices. The bleeding may occur after a period of upper respiratory symptoms and coughing. Management is initially conservative with sedation and bedrest; surgery ir rarely needed.
   b. Esophagitis-this is a result of persistent gastroesophageal reflux leading to inflammation and generally slow, chronic loss of blood from the weeping mucosa. Treatment consist of antacids, frequent small feeds, occasionally medications and if not rapidly improved, then surgical intervention with a fundoplication ofthe stomach.
   c. Mallory-Weiss-this is a tear of the distal esophagus and/or gastroesophageal junction secondary to severe regurgitation. This was thought to be uncommon in children because it was not looked for by endoscopy. It probably occurs more often than previously thought. Treatment initially is conservative and, if persistent, oversewing of the tear through an incision in the stomach will be successful.
   d. Duplication cysts- Rare cause, they are seen on the mesenteric side of the intestine anywhere from the esophagus to the anus. They bleed when there is ectopic gastric mucosa present. Total excision is curative.
2. Stomach
   a. Gastric Erosions- managed medically in most cases.
   b. Ulcer- treated medically unless there is persistent hemorrhage, obstruction or perforation.

c. Hematoma- usually secondary to trauma or bleeding disorders.

3. Duodenum
   a. Duodenitis- associated to acid peptic disease.
   b. Hematobilia- secondary to blunt or penetrating abdominal injury. Occasionally requires surgical intervention with local repair or ligation of hepatic vessels.

Lower GI bleeding (Older Children)

Anal Fissure

Anal fissure is the most common cause of rectal bleeding in the first two years of life. Outstretching of the anal mucocutaneous junction caused by passage of large hard stools during defecation produces a superficial tear of the mucosa in the posterior midline. Pain with the next bowel movement leads to constipation, hardened stools that continue to produce cyclic problems. Large fissures with surrounding bruising should warn against child abuse. Crohn's disease and leukemic infiltration are other conditions to rule-out. The diagnosis is made after inspection of the anal canal. Chronic fissures are associated with hypertrophy of the anal papilla or a distal skin tag. Management is directed toward the associated constipation with stool softeners and anal dilatations, warm perineal baths to relax the internal muscle spasm, and topical analgesics for pain control. If medical therapy fails excision of the fissure with lateral sphincterotomy is performed.

Meckel's Diverticulum

Meckel's diverticulum denotes those anatomic structures resulting from the umbilical and intra-abdominal persistence of the embryonic vitelline duct (yolk stalk). Meckel's diverticulum is clinically significant, either when discovered incidentally at celiotomy or recognize as the cause of symptoms, which are intestinal bleeding, abdominal pain, or intestinal obstruction. Children with symptomatic Meckel's present with hemorrhage (40%), intestinal obstruction (30%), diverticulitis (20%), and umbilical discharge or disease (6%). Diagnosis is related to presentation. Intermittent rectal bleeding may be diagnosed on occasion **by 99mTc sodium pertechtenate**. Barium studies are unreliable. Persistent bleeding requires laparotomy even if the Meckel's scan is negative. Diverticulitis or perforation presents with finding similar to appendicitis. Obstruction secondary to intussusception is diagnosed by clinical findings and barium enema. Incidental Meckel's diverticulum is generally handled by simple wedge excision in children. Bleeding Meckel's is managed by resection of the bowel and end-to-end anastomosis. Diverticulitis is handled by either method. Asymptomatic Meckel's diverticula identified incidentally should be removed if upon palpation there is questionable ectopic (gastric or pancreatic) mucosa.

Polyps

Juvenile Polyps comprise 80% of childhood polyps. This is a **mucous retention polyp** and histologically features a cluster of mucoid lobes surrounded by flattened mucus-secreting glandular cells. There is **no malignant potential**. These polyps are most commonly seen in children age 3-10 with a peak at age 5-6. 85% of children have a solitary polyp. The most common complaint is rectal bleeding and occasionally the polyps may prolapse out the rectum. Diagnosis is by barium enema, rectal exam and/or endoscopy. Removal by endoscopy is the treatment of choice. rarely, exploratory lap with colotomy and excision is required. Lymphoid polyps are not polyps at all, but rather localized elevations of colonic mucosa that on barium enema produce filling defects resembling polyps. They are produced by hyperplasia of submucosal lymphoid tissue. These make up about 15% of childhood polyps. They begin to appear during the first year of life, peak at about the third year of life, and diminish in number by 5 years of age. These are multiple and may present with mild chronic blood loss. Diagnosis is made by barium enema. endoscopy and biopsy. No treatment is necessary since they will regress spontaneously. Peutz-Jeghers syndrome are polyps associated with melanin hyperpigmentation of the lips and oral mucosa. The polyps are usually multiple and hamartomas. They will appear anywhere, but the majority are limited to the jejunum and ileum. Chronic blood loss anemia in a child with repeated bouts of colicky abdominal pain secondary to actual or incipient intussusception are typical. Diagnosis is by contrast studies. GI malignancy has been reported in 2-3% of patients. Females with Peutz-Jeghers syndrome seem predisposed to develop ovarian tumors, usually in adolescence. Treatment depends on the severity of symptoms and extend of involvement. Familial Polyposis Coli has an autosomal dominant inheritance. Hundreds of adenomatous colonic polyps with virtually all developing adenocarcinoma of colon by the third decade of life. The most common and best-recognized variant is patients with Gardner's syndrome, which combines the premalignant adenomatous colonic polyps with soft and hard tissue tumors. Diagnosis is by family history, and contrast studies followed by biopsy. Treatment is total colectomy with ileostomy or endorectal pull-through with ileo-anal anastomosis.

Familial Adenomatous Polyposis (FAP)

Familial history of colon cancer is an important indicator of future risk for colorectal cancer. The more extensive and closer the affected relatives, the greater the risk. Highest risk is found in Familial Adenomatous Polyposis (FAP). Once the risk is appreciated screening for the disease must take place. This involves genetic analysis for members of syndrome families along with lower gastrointestinal endoscopy for the rest as polyps can occur throughout the gastrointestinal tract. FAP is a genetic (autosomal dominant) premalignant condition that will ultimately manifest with the development of colorectal carcinoma. FAP has been linked to germline mutations of the adenomatous polyposis coli (APC) gene. Initial presentation can be rectal bleeding. Besides multiple adenomatous polyps of the colon predisposing to malignancy at an early age, a variety of extra colonic manifestations are associated with this condition. Once the diagnosis of FAP is established endoscopic surveillance should be instituted. **All polyps should be subjected to histopathological exam to determine presence of adenomatous epithelium**. With the presence of dysplastic changes total colectomy with the creation of an ileorectal or ileoanal (pouch) anastomosis is recommended. Almost one-third of cases develops adenomas in the ileal pouch after proctocolectomy. Baseline small bowel enteroscopy should be done at the time of surgery and in the postop period in children with FAP and juvenile polyposis. With duodenal polyps enteroscopy should be done at the time of surgery. Biopsy and/or excision of larger polyps should be done as they may harbor a carcinoma.

PANCREATIC, HEPATIC, BILIARY AND SPLENIC DISORDERS

Annular Pancreas/Pancreas Divisum

The pancreas develops from an anterior and posterior anlage of the foregut early during gestation (28days). The anterior bud leads to the liver and body and tail of the pancreas. The posterior diverticulum develops into the head of the pancreas. This bud rotates anteriorly and later fuses to achieve the relationship to the rest of the pancreas . Under the influence of this mesenchyme the mature organ develops, being mainly composed of ductal, exocrine and endocrine cells. Exocrine and ductal pancreas are derived from the endoderm of the foregut. Recent evidence suggests that the endocrine cells derive also from the endoderm of the foregut as evidenced by the expression of the genes responsible for hormonal production. This challenges the theory that endocrine cells may originate from the neural crest cells (neuroectodermal) of the embryo reinforced by the enunciation of the amine precursor uptake decarboxylase (APUD) theory.

Annular pancreas is the most common congenital malformation of the pancreas in association with duodenal atresia. Embryologically the ring formation (annulus) originates from the ventral pancreas primordium . The pancreatic duct of the annular tissue passed from the anterior portion to the lateral and posterior portion finally joining with the main pancreatic duct. Two types of annular pancreas are recognized:

1. *Extramural:* causing high gastrointestinal obstruction; vomiting is the most common presenting symptom,and
2. *Intramural:* producing duodenal ulceration. Presentation at birth is affected by the degree of duodenal obstruction and coexistent anomalies. Polyhydramnios usually accompanies complete high intestinal obstruction in annular pancreas. Associated anomalies can range from malrotation, intrinsic duodenal obstruction, Down syndrome and duodenal bands. ERCP is the most important procedure to find the characteristic features and establish the therapeutic strategy in cases of annular pancreas. Experience militates against any direct attack on the offending annulus. Therefore, all children with this abnormality are generally treated with a bypass procedure, preferably a duodeno-duodenostomy. Long-term complications may include cholestatic jaundice, upper gastrointestinal motility disorder, failure to thrive, chronic diarrhea and chronic relapsing pancreatitis due to an incomplete divisum anomaly. Pancreas divisum (PD), believed the most common congenital anomaly of the pancreas, is an embryologic variation of pancreas development where the dorsal (Santorini) and ventral portions (Wirsung) ducts drain

separately. Diagnosis is made with ERCP (short duct of Wirsung that does not communicate with main pancreatic duct of Santorini). Not everybody with this ductal anomaly develops pancreatitis. Likewise with the minor papilla draining the bulk of the pancreas in PD, a small orifice size (< 0.75 mm) plays a role in outflow obstruction and development of pancreatitis. Children with PD and recurrent episodes of pancreatitis will need endoscopic sphincterotomy of the minor and sometimes major papilla. If not feasible technically, surgical sphincteroplasty of both papillae along with cholecystectomy (bile stasis leads to gallstones) is indicated. Intraoperative pancreatogram will help determine if both papilla are stenotic. Once chronic pancreatitis is established, ductal drainage or resection may be necessary.

Pancreatitis

Acute pancreatitis (AP) is unusual in the pediatric patient, can affect all age groups and should be considered in children presenting with acute abdominal complaints.Causes are diversely and clinical course less severe. The three most common etiological factors are: trauma, drug-induced, and biliary tract disorders.Other factors to consider are: infections (mumps, ascaris, adenovirus), metabolic (branched-chain organic acidemias), structural defects (anomalous union of pancreatico-biliary ductal system), and hereditary. Blunt abdominal trauma is the leading cause (20-30%)of AP by crushing the fixed organ between the spine. Drugs associated to the development of AP are: steroids, L-asparaginase, valproic acid, acetaminophen (drug withdrawal is treatment of choice). Biliary disorders related to AP are gallstone and choledochal cysts by causing transient ductal obstruction. Most common complaint of children with AP is abdominal pain. Diagnosis is confirmed with elevated amylase/lipase in serum and urine (lipase is more specific since pancreas is major source). Imaging studies of utility are US, CT-Scan and ERCP. The use of ERCP in previously idiopathic cases of AP have increased the yield of diagnosing anomalous pancreatico-biliary junctional defects. Management during early phase is supportive with IV therapy, NG decompression, NPO (to decrease acid stimulation and prevent secretin release), and nutritional (TPN). Surgery is rarely required except complications such as abscess and pseudocyst formation. Uncommon disorder in childhood. Trauma (compressed injury against spinal column) and biliary tract disorders (choledochal cyst, cholelithiasis) are most common cause of pancreatitis. The most common congenital ductal anomaly leading to pancreatitis is pancreas divisum. Most common complaint is midepigastric abdominal trauma associated with nausea and vomiting. Diagnosis is confirmed with elevated levels of amylase and lipase. Ultrasound is useful to determine degree of edema and presence of pseudocyst formation. Treatment consists of: NPO, NG decompression, decrease acid stimulation (H-2 blockers), aprotinin, glucagon, and anticholinergics. Pain is relieved with meperidine. When pancreatic serum enzymes level return to near normal level patient is started in low-fat diet. Antibiotic prophylaxis use is controversial. Surgery is indicated for: abscess formation and pseudocyst. Pseudocysts are the result of major ductal disruptions or minor lacerations. Observation allows spontaneous resolution in 40-60% of cases. Percutaneous aspiration and catheter drainage is another alternative in management. Follow-up studies permit determine if cavity is decreasing in size. This can be done outpatient teaching parents to irrigate the catheter at home to assure patency. Persistency beyond 6 months may need resectional therapy. Additional option is internal drainage (cyst-gastrostomy, cyst-jejunostomy). Abscess should be drained and debride. Pancreatic pseudocyst formation is an uncommon complication of pancreatic inflammatory disease (pancreatitis) or trauma in children. More than half cases are caused by blunt abdominal trauma. Ultrasound is the most effective and non-invasive way of diagnosing pancreatic pseudocysts. Acute pseudocysts are managed expectantly for 4-6 wk. until spontaneous resolution occurs. 25-50% will undergo spontaneous resolution. Medical therapy consists of decreasing pancreatic stimulation and giving nutritional support. Rupture is the major complication of conservative management.

Chronic pseudocysts (> three month) will benefit from prompt operation and internal drainage since resolution is rare. Percutaneous catheter drainage under local anesthesia using Ultrasound or CT guided technique is an appropriate method of first-line therapy for non-resolving (chronic) or enlarging pancreatic pseudocysts. The approach is transgastric or transcutaneous.

Those cysts that fail to resolve with percutaneous drainage should go investigation of ductal anatomy to rule out disruption of the main pancreatic duct. The need for further surgery (drainage or resectional) will depend on the status of the duct of Wirsung.

Pancreatic Cysts

Pancreatic cystic lesions are usually inflammatory pseudocyst (90%) or neoplastic process (10%). Distinguishing between them is essential for appropriate surgical therapy. Non-inflammatory neoplastic cysts in children are very rare ductal lesions with a spectrum of histologic characteristics and favorable outcomes. Histologically they include retention cysts, lymphoepithelial cysts, papillary cystic tumors, benign serous cystadenoma, mucinous tumors and mucinous cystadenocarcinoma. Most reported cases occur in females during adolescent years. Mode of presentation includes mild upper abdominal pain and palpable mass. Clinical, radiographic and intraoperative frozen section are non-reliable methods in distinguishing the different types of pancreatic cysts.

Preoperative cyst fluid obtained by US or CT-guided percutaneous aspiration can be analyzed for viscosity (mucoid, viscous, serous), chemical (amylase, lipase), tumor markers (CEA, CA 19-9, CA125) and cytology characteristics. High CEA levels (> 25 ng/ml) indicate that the cyst is either malignant or mucinous (premalignant) type. Higher levels of CA 19-9 suggest pseudocysts and serous cystadenomas. Very high CA 125 levels appear predictive of malignancy. Viscosity above 1.63 suggests mucinous tumors. Amylase and lipase content should be low in true pancreatic cysts. Cytology analysis is insensitive unless positive for tumor cells. When the nature of the pancreatic cyst cannot be definitively establish by the above methods surgical resection is indicated.

Hepatic Cysts

Hepatic cysts (HC) can be either parasitic (echinococcal) following infestation in endemic regions, acquired (after trauma or inflammatory processes), or nonparasitic (congenital) in nature. Congenital nonparasitic HC are uncommon, solitary, benign lesions that arise from aberrant development of intrahepatic biliary radicals after ischemic thrombo-embolic phenomena (vascular disruption theory). The cyst is lined with cuboidal or squamous epithelium, and there is a female and white children predominance. Although generally asymptomatic, children may manifest increased abdominal girth, vague abdominal discomfort, infection, or obstructive jaundice. Ultrasound and CT-Scan are diagnostic tools. Management may consist of: simple unroofing, complete removal by enucleation or hepatic lobectomy, internal Roux-en-Y drainage, or percutaneous aspiration and sclerosis (alcohol, minocycline). The surgical alternative to use will depend on size, location (central, peripheral or dumbbell), and presence of communication with biliary system of the cyst . Some cases diagnosed prenatally or during the neonatal period have undergone slow spontaneous regression.

Biliary Atresia

Persistent conjugated hyperbilirubinemia (greater than 20% of total or 1.5 mg%) should be urgently evaluated. Initial evaluation should include a well-taken history and physical exam, partial and total bilirubin determination, type and blood group, Coomb's test, reticulocyte cell count and a peripheral smear. Cholestasis means a reduction in bile flow in the liver, which depends on the biliary excretion of the conjugated portion. Reduce flow causes retention of biliary lipoproteins that stimulates hypercholesterolemia causing progressive damage to the hepatic cell, fibrosis, cirrhosis and altered liver function tests. **Biliary Atresia (BA) is the most common cause of persistently direct (conjugated) hyperbilirubinemia in the first three months of life**. It is characterized by progressive inflammatory obliteration of the extrahepatic bile ducts, an estimated incidence of one in 15,000 live births, and predominance of female patients. The disease is the result of an acquired inflammatory process with gradual degeneration of the epithelium of the extrahepatic biliary ducts causing luminal obliteration, cholestasis, and biliary cirrhosis. The timing of the insult after birth suggests a viral etiology obtained transplacentally. Almost 20% of patients have associated anomalies such as: polysplenia, malrotation, situs inversus, pre-duodenal portal vein and absent inferior vena cava. Histopathology is distinguished by an inflammatory process in several dynamic stages with progressive destruction, scar formation, and chronic granulation tissue of bile ducts. Physiologic jaundice of the newborn is a common, benign, and self-limiting condition. In BA the patient develops insidious jaundice by the second week of life. The baby looks active, not acutely ill and progressively develops acholic stools, choluria and hepatomegaly. Non-surgical source of cholestasis shows a sick, low weight infant who is jaundiced since birth. The diagnostic evaluation of the cholestatic infant should include a series of lab tests that can exclude perinatal infectious (TORCH titers, hepatitis profile), metabolic (alpha-1-antitrypsin levels), systemic and hereditary causes. Total bilirubin in BA babies is around 6-10 mg%, with 50-80% conjugated. Liver function tests are nonspecific. Lipoprotein-X levels greater than 300 mg% and Gamma Glutamyl Transpeptidase (GGT) above 200 units% suggest the diagnosis. The presence of the yellow bilirubin pigment in the aspirate of duodenal content excludes the diagnosis of BA. Ultrasound study of the abdomen should be the first diagnostic imaging study done to cholestatic infants to evaluate the presence of a gallbladder, identify intra or extrahepatic bile ducts dilatation, and liver parenchyma echogenicity. The postprandial contraction of the gallbladder eliminates the possibility of BA even when nuclear studies are positive. **Nuclear studies of bilio-enteric excretion (DISIDA) after pre-stimulation of the microsomal hepatic system with phenobarbital for 3-5 days is the diagnostic imaging test of choice**. The presence of the radio-isotope in the GI tract excludes the diagnosis of BA. Percutaneous liver biopsy should be the next diagnostic step. The mini-laparotomy is the final diagnostic alternative. Those infant with radiographic evidence of patent extrahepatic biliary tract has no BA. Medical management of BA is uniformly fatal. Kasai portoenterostomy has decreased the mortality of BA during the last 30 years. Kasai procedure consists of removing the obliterated extrahepatic biliary system, and anastomosing the most proximal part to a bowel segment. Almost three-fourth of patients will develop portal hypertension in spite of adequate postoperative bile flow. They will manifest esophageal varices, hypersplenism, and ascites. Hepatic transplantation is reserved for those patients with failed portoenterostomy, progressive liver failure or late-referral to surgery.

Biliary Hypoplasia

Biliary hypoplasia is a rare cause of persistent neonatal conjugated hyperbilirubinemia. Pathologically, affected children have absent or reduced number of bile ductules with normal distribution of branches of the portal vein and hepatic artery within the liver parenchyma. Biliary hypoplasia is also identified as paucity of interlobular bile ducts (PILBD). Two types of PILBD are recognized: 1) syndromic (arteriohepatic dysplasia or Alagille's syndrome) with characteristic extrahepatic abnormalities (fascial appearance, pulmonic artery stenosis, vertebral anomalies, embryotoxon and delayed weight-height development), and 2) non-syndromic biliary hypoplasia. Biliary hypoplasia is clinically indistinguishable from biliary atresia and can sometimes be confused. **A definitive diagnosis is difficult to make in early infancy. Differentiation between biliary atresia, hypoplasia and neonatal hepatitis continues to require direct visualization of the biliary ducts. This mean laparoscopic or open intra-operative cholangiography and liver biopsy.** The cholangiogram will show diminutive intra- and extra-hepatic biliary tree. Attempts to establish biliary flow by means of hepatic porto-enterostomy (Kasai procedures) in children with PILBD have been unsuccessful and contraindicated. Management is conservative and include predigested formulas, ursodeoxycholic acids (10 mg/kg/day), phenobarbital and A,D,K,E vitamin replacement. Non-syndromic PILBD have better long-term prognosis. Children with syndromic PILBD identified in infancy because of cholestasis have a 50% probability of long-term survival without liver transplantation.

Choledochal Cyst

Choledochal cyst is a rare dilatation of the common bile duct, prevalent in oriental patients (Japan), where >60% of patients are less than 10 years old. The etiology is related to an abnormal pancreatic-biliary junction (common channel theory) causing reflux of pancreatic enzymes into the common bile duct (trypsin and amylase). Symptoms are: abdominal pain, obstructive jaundice, a palpable abdominal mass, cholangitis, and pancreatitis. Infants develop jaundice more frequently, causing diagnostic problems with Biliary Atresia. Older children may show abdominal pain and mass. Jaundice is less severe and intermittent. Diagnosis is confirmed with Ultrasound and corroborated with a HIDA (or DISIDA) Scan. Choledochal cysts are classified depending on morphology and localization. Management is surgical and consist of cyst excision and Roux-en-Y hepaticojejunostomy reconstruction. Cyst retention penalties paid are: stricture, cholangitis, stone formation, pancreatitis, biliary cirrhosis, and malignancy. Long-term follow-up after surgery is advised.

SpienicCyst, Splenoptosis, Spherocytosis and Asplenia

Splenic cysts in children are either considered true epidermal (congenital), pseudocysts (post-traumatic), or infectious (echinococcus) in etiology. They are rare, benign, solitary cysts often producing few symptoms. They may present as a palpable mass in the left side of the abdomen or during evaluation for another abdominal problem. Ultrasound (large unilocular sonolucent cyst) is the most important diagnostic method, and can be supplemented by CT-Scan. The lining of the cyst is a flattened endothelium surrounded by fibrous tissue. This mesothelium can produced carcinoembryonic antigen (CEA). Indications for surgery are: (i) risk of complications (rupture, bleeding), (ii) size greater than 5 cm., (iii) infectious etiology, and a (iv) symptomatic child (pain, mass or splenomegaly). Their management formerly total splenectomy has changed to: interventional sonography with fluid aspiration (catheter placement), or partial splenic decapsulation (cystectomy); the result of recognition of the physiologic importance (hematologic and immunologic) of the spleen, together with the development of radiological imaging and operative surgery. Long term follow-up with radionuclide scans is recommended.

Splenoptosis (Wandering spleen) is a rare congenital fusion anomaly of the dorsal mesogastrium of the spleen that results in failure and laxity of its normal attachment to the diaphragm, retroperitoneum and colon. Relatively more common in children than adults, and females outnumber males. The child presents with an asymptomatic mass (splenomegaly), mass and subacute gastrointestinal complaints or with acute abdominal symptoms. These are the result of torsion of the pedicle, ischemia and splenic sequestration. 50% of spleens are lost to acute ischemia from torsion. Other complications are: pancreatitis, hypersplenism and cyst formation. Lab tests are nonspecific, but may occasionally reveal evidence of hypersplenism or functional asplenia. Diagnosis needs a high index of suspicion, and is achieved with: Ultrasound, CT, and Scintigram. Management consists of splenectomy for frank splenic infarct, or splenopexy for viable organs. Splenopexy is achieved by creating an extraperitoneal pocket or wrapping the spleen in absorbable mesh and anchoring to the retroperitoneum

Hereditary spherocytosis is a clinically heterogenous autosomal dominant red blood cell membrane disorder that causes anemia. The genetic defect results in deficiency of spectrin, the largest and most abundant structural protein of the erythrocyte membrane skeleton. The affected RBC loses its biconcave shape, strength and flexibility to the stress of circulation, becomes round and is trapped and destructs early in the spleen. Initial symptoms are those of pallor, jaundice and chronic anemia, followed by splenomegaly. Hemolytic crises are triggered by intercurrent infections. Pigment gallstones are common after the first decade of life. Labs' findings are those of many spherocytes in the peripheral smear, 8-10 mg% hemoglobin, elevated reticulocyte count, increase erythropoiesis in the bone marrow, and negative Coomb's test. Erythrocytes' shows increased osmotic fragility with autohemolysis in hypotonic solutions. Definitive therapy consists of splenectomy. **This condition is the most common indication for elective splenectomy in children**. The risk of overwhelming postsplenectomy sepsis makes it advisable to delay splenectomy until after six years of age unless the child becomes transfusion dependent. At the time of splenectomy, it is important to identify and remove accessory spleens. If gallstones are present, cholecystectomy should be done. A low content of spectrin and high percentage of microcyte has been used as determinants of early splenectomy as judge by the clinical severity of the disease process. Howell-Jolly bodies in erythrocyte are identified after total splenectomy. The absence of the spleen (asplenia) occurs after surgical removal, following chronic conditions or congenital. **Trauma is the most common cause of removing the spleen in children and sickle cell disease is the most common cause of functional asplenia in children.** Asplenia increases the risk of fulminant bacteremia (post-splenectomy sepsis) and mortality with these organisms. This risk is also increased by the underlying condition that caused the removal of the spleen, i.e., trauma, malignancy or hematologic disease. Several recommendations have been given when dealing with an asplenic individual. These are to vaccinate the child against pneumococcus (Pneumovax vaccine), hemophilus influenza type b and meningococcus. Regarding Pneumovax use revaccination after 3-5 years is recommended for children with asplenia who are 10 years of age or younger and for older children and adults who were immunized at least five years before. Duration of vaccine-induced antibodies is unknown but may be shorter than that in normal persons. Long-term antimicrobial prophylaxis is also used. This carries the problem of compliance and for how long. Significant febrile episodes should be managed aggressively, and probably most important, the patient and family should be carefully educated about this complication (name tag). Most deaths from hyposplenia-related septicemia are preventable.

Splenic Trauma

Spleen is the most common injured organ in blunt abdominal trauma. Hematologic and immunologic importance of the spleen has changed the attitude of trauma surgeons toward preservation of this organ whenever hemodynamics physiology permits. Massive hemorrhage (> 50 cc/kg weight) and hemodynamic instability are indications for surgery. CT-Scan continues to be the choice of imaging during blunt abdominal trauma to establish the diagnosis of solid organ rupture in blunt abdominal trauma and rule out other major abdominal injuries. Isolated splenic rupture can be managed conservative in almost 80-90% of cases reducing complications and post-splenectomy sepsis. Low velocity of injury, thicker capsule, ribs elasticity and transverse nature of the laceration explain propensity for spontaneous healing in children. Associated lesions are not a contraindication for conservative management. Should conservative management fails the next step is splenography or splenectomy. Child is admitted to intensive care for 48 hours, followed by in-hospital observation until stable to be discharge home. Vaccination (pneumococcus, hemophilus and meningococci) affords added protection. Sonography is helpful for sequential splenic imaging to show when the appearance returns to normal, though clinical exam suffices. Participation in body contact sports should be curtailed for at least three months after injury.

TUMORS

Wilms Tumor

This is the most common solid intra-abdominal tumor (malignant) in children. Neuroblastoma is most common, but they are not all confined to the abdomen. It has a peak incidence at 3-5 years of age. Present as abdominal or flank mass with abdominal pain, asymptomatic hematuria, and occasionally fever. Other presentations: malaise, weight loss, anemia, left varicocele (obstructed left renal vein), hypertension. Abnormalities associated with Wilms tumor include hemihypertrophy, pseudohermaphroditism, aniridia, Beckwith-Wiedemann syndrome, trisomy 18 and other genitourinary anomalies. The initial evaluation consist of: abdominal films, ultrasound, IVP, urinalysis, and chest-X-rays and tomography. The presence of a solid, intrarenal mass causing intrinsic distortion of the calyceal collecting system is virtually diagnostic of Wilms tumor. Sonography can be of help to evaluate the IVC and renal veins (venous extension of the tumor). Metastasis most common in the lung and occasionally the liver. Operation is for both treatment and staging to determine further therapy. The abdomen is explored by a large transverse incision and both kidneys are visualized. Nodes are biopsied to determine extent of disease.

Staging by National Wilms Tumor Study Group:

Group I: tumor limited to kidney and completely resected.

Group II: tumor extends beyond the kidney but is completely excised.

Group III: residual non-hematogenous tumor confined to the abdomen.

Group IV: hematogenous metastasis.

Group V: bilateral tumors.

Further treatment with chemotherapy or radiotherapy depends on staging and histology (favorable vs non-favorable) of tumor. Non-favorable histologic characteristics are: anaplasia (enlarged nucleus 3X, hyperchromatism, mitosis), sarcomatous or rhabdoid degeneration.

Disease-free survival is 95% for Stage I and approximately 77% for all patients. Poor prognosis for those with lymph nodes, lung and liver metastasis.

Neuroblastoma

Neuroblastoma is the most common solid tumor of infancy and childhood. Most appear during the first five years of life; over half occur in children under 2 years of age. Two-thirds of children over 2 years of age have disseminated disease at presentation.

Neuroblastomas can occur at any site where neural crest tissue is found in the embryo and are derived from primordial neural crest cells and neuroblasts migrating from the mantle layer of the developing spinal cord into the sympathetic ganglion chain and the adrenal medulla. The etiology is unknown. About three-fourths of neuroblastomas arise in the abdomen; half of these originate in the adrenal gland. About 20% occur in the posterior mediastinum. Other uncommon sites include the pelvis (4%), and the neck (4%). It's a solid, highly vascular tumor with a friable pseudocapsule.

Staging

Stage I: tumor limited to organ of origin.
Stage II: regional spread that does not cross the midline.

Stage III: tumor extending across the midline.

Stage IV: distant metastasis.

Stage IV: S patients with a small primary and metastases limited to liver, skin, or bone marrow without radiographic evidence of bone metastases.

The clinical presentation is an abdominal mass (50-75%), hypertension (25%), weight loss, diarrhea, fever, bone pain. Rare: "opso-myoclonus" (dancing eye syndrome), Horner's syndrome, Panda's eyes, VIP syndromes.

Diagnostic work-up includes: IVP, ultrasound, chest films, KUB (fine stipple calcifications 50%), skull x-rays, urinalysis, CBC, Urine VMA, HVA, and bone marrow aspirate. Other markers: cystathione, homoserine, neuron-specific enolase and ferritin.

The surgical goal is complete removal of the tumor when possible. Unfortunately, metastases are present in 60-90% of patients at diagnosis. Even in these patients attempts to reduce the bulk of tumor is important. Further treatment with radiation and chemotherapy depends on stage and extent of metastases.

There is a 100% survival for stage I, although this stage is extremely rare. Survival for stage II is 75%, stage III is 35%, stage IV 10-20%, and stage IV-S is about 80%. Age is an important prognostic factor, with 75% survival in children less than one year; 50% in children 1-2 years of age; 25% in children 2-3 years of age, and 15% in children over 3 years. Other prognostic factors are related to stage, nutritional status, site of primary, maturity state of tumor, VIP tumor (+), positive lymph nodes (-), high ferritin, NSE, and Diploid DNA levels(-).

Routine use of prenatal sonography will increase the incidental diagnosis of fetal neuroblastoma. Most are detected during the third trimester of pregnancy as cystic/solid suprarenal mass. **The tumor does not cross the placenta but can metastasize in utero to the fetal liver or placenta**. After birth 50% of babies have elevated HMA/VMA levels. Most enjoy improved survival due to: lower stage of disease, cystic variety (in-situ), and higher stage IV-S (which has been associated with spontaneous immuno-regression. Adverse biologic features are: diploid tumor karyotype (cytometry) and amplify N-myc oncogene. They can be very difficult to differentiate from neonatal adrenal hemorrhage; T2 of MRI can be of help. Are they neuroblastoma in-situ, and will they regress spontaneously without treatment are question waiting answer in the near future. Neuroblastoma (NB) in early stages of development (stage I & II) benefits from surgical excision. The role of surgery in the management of neuroblastoma stage III tumor (tumor infiltrating across the midline with or without lymph node involvement) is controversial. Many variables enter the formula of determining risk of disease, i.e., age, site, stage, N-myc status, DNA diploidy and Shimada classification to mention a few of the most important. Some reports have independently found that stage III managed initially with chemotherapy and radiotherapy and is responding benefits from eventual complete tumor excision despite site, age or histology. Complete surgical excision as determine by free margin of tissue has a significant survival advantage overall. Preop chemotx converts a friable tumor into a firmer, more mature and easily resectable tumor. Surgical complications in advance stages are higher (bleeding, nephrectomy, adjacent organ removal, infection). Biologically unfavorable patients one year of age or greater who undergo gross surgical resections has improved survival. Defining subgroups of patient with poor prognostic biologic markers and histology to decide whether surgery or bone marrow transplant is the next best option is pending trial randomization and study. Stage IV Neuroblastoma (metastatic NB) refers to high risk group of children with the primary tumor in the adrenal gland, mediastinum or pelvis associated with disease progression in other sites (bone marrow, cortical bone, liver, lymph node). Role of surgery in stage IV NB is controversial. Cure will require control of the primary tumor and elimination of metastatic disease. For infants with metastatic NB a more than 95% resection has been found adequate surgical treatment either initially or after effective chemotherapy. Adding ipsilateral lymph node dissection does not appear to affect survival. Delayed surgery after several courses of chemotherapy may be as effective as initial resection and is associated with fewer complications statistically.

Resection without induct on chemotherapy result in significant blood loss. High risk NB usually invades blood vessels and surrounding structures precluding resection. Intensive preoperative

Therapy reduces tumor size and invasiveness allowing surgical removal. A fibrotic capsule forms with less blood supply to the tumor. Stage IV tumor is best managed with chemotherapy. Gross complete resection is best accomplished when a good partial response is obtained .

Resection is not confounded by biology of the tumor (n-myc status). Survival is improved with kidney preservation during surgery. Local control of disease is a prerequisite for successful bone marrow transplantation.

Rhabdomyosarcoma

Most common soft tissue sarcoma in infants and children and represents about 5-15% of all solid malignant lesions. It has a peak incidence at age 2-5 years. Second surge between 10-15 years of age. Tumors of the pelvic organs and head and neck are more prevalent in infancy and early childhood, while the paratesticular rhabdomyosarcomas are largely a disease of adolescents and young adults. Although classically described as occurring in striated muscle, rhabdomyosarcomas arise from a primitive cell type and occur in mesenchymal tissue at almost any body site (possibly excluding the brain), including many organs that normally do not have striated muscle. The predominant histologic type in infants and small children is embryonal. The botryoid rhabdomyosarcoma is a subtype of the embryonal variety, which ordinarily extends into body cavities such as the bladder, nasopharynx, vagina, or bile duct. The alveolar cell type, named for a superficial resemblance to the pulmonary alveoli, is the most common form found on the muscle masses of the trunk and extremities, and is seen more frequently as age advances.

The clinical findings, diagnostic evaluation and therapy employed are dependent upon the location of the primary tumor and is beyond the scope of this review. In brief, head and neck tumors are most common and occur in the orbit, nasopharynx, cheek, neck, middle ear, larynx and paranasal sinuses. Most are treated by simple biopsy followed by combined therapy or preoperative chemotherapy and radiation followed by conservative resection. Operations for extremity lesions include wide local excision to remove as much of the gross tumor as possible. Rhabdomyosarcomas can arise from the bladder, prostate, uterus, or vagina. The trend in treatment is more chemotherapy and conservative surgical management.

Liver Tumors

Hepatoblastoma and hepatocellular carcinoma are the most common malignant tumor of liver. These represent about 2% of all malignancies in childhood and 15% of malignant abdominal masses. Hepatoblastoma (HB) is the most common primary malignant neoplasm of the liver in children mostly seen in males less than four year of age. Diagnostic work-up (US, Scintigraphy, CT-Scan) objective is predicting resectability and tumor extension. Diagnostic laparotomy will decide resectability. Markers associated to this tumor are: alpha-fetoprotein and gamma-glutamyltransferase II. Only reliable chances of cure is surgical excision . Hepatocellular carcinoma in childhood is histologically identical to hepatoma seen in the adult and is associated 50% of the time to a prior liver disorder (i.e. tyrosinemia, hepatitis type B, etc.).

Associated anomalies and conditions are: hemihypertrophy, osteoporosis, lipid storage disease, glycogen storage disease, virilization in males. Clinical presentation is asymptomatic abdominal mass, with abdominal pain and weight loss in 25% of patients. Diagnostic work-up includes: alpha-fetoprotein, chest x-ray, abdominal films, IVP, ultrasound, liver spleen scan, CAT scan, and occasionally arteriogram. Hepatic resection has provided the only cures. In patients with initially unresectable tumor or in postresection patients, chemotherapy is employed. Among those patients in whom the entire tumor can be resected, survival is 80% at two years. Unresectable tumors have a dismal prognosis. ADR (adriamycin) is the principal chemotherapeutic agent.

Teratomas

Teratomas contains tissues derived from the three embryonic layers (endoderm, mesoderm, and ectoderm), found in a locus that does not normally harbor such tissues. It is not always possible to find tissue in each teratoma that is derived from all three embryonic layers. Sacrococcygeal teratoma (SCT) is the most common extragonadal germ cell tumor in neonates with an incidence of one in 30-40,000 live births. Three-fourth are females. SCT present as a large, firm or more commonly cystic masses that arise from the anterior surface of the sacrum or coccyx, protruding and forming a large external mass. Histology consist of tissue from the three germ cell layers. SCT is classified as: mature, immature, or malignant (endodermal sinus) and produces alpha-feto protein (AFP). Prenatal sonographic diagnostic severity criteria are: tumor size greater than the biparietal diameter of the fetus, rapid tumor growth, development of placentomegaly, polyhydramnios and hydrops. Large tumors should benefit from cesarean section to avoid dystocia or tumor rupture. Management consist of total tumor resection with coccyx (recurrence is associated with leaving coccyx in place). Every recurrence of SCT should be regarded as potentially malignant. Malignant or immature SCT with elevated AFP after surgical resection will benefit from adjuvant chemotherapy. Survival is 95% for mature/immature tumors, but less than 80% for malignant cases. Follow-up should consist of (i) meticulous physical exam every 3-6 months for first three years, (ii) serial AFP determination, (iii) fecal/urodynamic functional studies. Long term F/U has found a 40% incidence of fecal and urinary impairment associated to either tumor compression of pelvic structures or surgical trauma.

Burkitt's Lymphoma

Burkitt's lymphoma (BL) is a highly malignant tumor first described during the late 50's in African children (jaw), endemic in nature, and composed of undifferentiated lympho-reticular cells with uniform appearance. The American BL variety is non-endemic, mostly attacks children between 8-12 years of age,predominantly (>75%) with abdominal disease such as unexplained mass, pain, or intussusception. The head and neck region follows. The tumor can appear as a localized, diffuse (multifocal, non-resectable) or metastatic abdominal mass (bone marrow and CNS). It's considered the fastest growing tumor in humans with a doubling time around 12-24 hrs. Chemotherapy is the primary treatment modality due to its effectiveness in rapidly proliferating cells. The role of surgery is to establish the diagnosis (using open biopsy), stage the tumor, remove localized disease, relieve intestinal obstruction and provide vascular access. Complete resection whenever possible offers the patient improved survival. Is more readily accomplished in patients with localized bowel involvement operated on an emergency basis due to acute abdominal symptoms. The only predictor of event free survival is extent of abdominal disease at diagnosis. Debulking (cytoreductive) procedures increases morbidity and delays initiation of chemotherapy worsening prognosis. Extensive tumors should be managed with minimal procedure and immediate chemotherapy (a/o radiotherapy). Bone marrow and CNS involvement are ominous prognostic signs.

GYNECOLOGIC AND INTERSEXUAL CONSIDERATIONS

Labial Adhesions in Infants

Minor labial adhesions is a common pediatric gynecologic problem occasionally confused with imperforate hymen. Most cases are in children 2-6 years old and involve labial adhesions secondary to diaper rash. The process causing fusion is a natural one: two normally covered surfaces with squamous epithelium in contact with each other is traumatized eventually forming a fibrous tissue union (agglutinate) between them when healing occurs. A small opening near the clitoris is always present through which urine escapes. This seldom causes symptoms except recurrent UTI if it covers the urethral meatus. Treatment consists of applying estrogenic creams (0.1%) for two weeks. Manual separation can be painful and adhesion recurs. Unless the urethral meatus is covered, there is no reason to be further aggressive in management. Prolonged use of estrogenic cream can cause precocious isosexual development.

Ovarian Cysts

Ovarian cysts in fetus and infants are usually follicular in nature and less than 2 cm in size. They are commonly diagnosed between the 28th and 39th wk. of gestation by sonography. Hypotheses on etiology are: (i) Excessive fetal gonadotropic activity, (ii) enzymatic abnormalities of the theca interna, and (iii) abnormal stimulation by the mother HCG. Obstetric management consists on observation and vaginal delivery. After birth, diagnostic assessment and management will depend on the size and sonographic characteristics of the cyst. Simple anechoic cysts, and those less than 5 cm in size can be observed for spontaneous resolution. Cyst with fluid debris, clot, septated or solid (complex nature), and larger than 5 cm should undergo surgical excision due to the higher incidence of torsion, perforation and hemorrhage associated to them. Percutaneous aspiration of large simple cysts with follow-up sonography is a well-accepted therapy, preserving surgery for recurrent or complicated cases. Surgical therapy is either cystectomy or oophorectomy that can result in loss of normal ovarian tissue.

Congenital Adrenal Hyperplasia

Congenital adrenal hyperplasia (CAH) involves a functional defect in any of the five enzymatic steps required for cortisol synthesis, most commonly 21-(involved in 90-95% of cases) and 11-hydroxylase level. This primary genetic defect transmitted as autosomal recessive impairs the ability of the adrenal cortex to synthesize cortisol causing increase feedback secretion of ACTH and adreno-cortical hyperplasia of the gland. Increase output of steroids proximal to the block (androgenic precursors) causes virilization in affected males and females. Its more severe form is associated with aldosterone deficiency and life-threatening salt wasting. Female pseudohermaphrodite due to virilizing CAH is the most frequent form of intersexuality found. The phenotypic picture varies from mild clitoral enlargement alone to complete masculinization of the urethral meatus at the tip of the penis. Prenatal diagnosis (southern blotting of DNA) is based on finding the disease gene on the short arm of chromosome 6. Likewise management in the mother (dexamethasone) is started empirically until the affected status is known by chorionic villus sampling. After birth management consists of cut-back or flap vaginoplasty with clitoral recession at 3-6 months of age. Children with high vaginal entry proximal to the urethra external sphincter can undergo early one-stage reconstruction at 8-12 months of age. Long term surgical results of female children show adequate sexual identification, reproduction, intellectual functioning and acceptable genitalia.

PRENATAL CONGENITAL MALFORMATIONS

Poor survival with neuroblastomas, diaphragmatic hernias and necrotizing enterocolitis requires efforts during the next few years to reduce mortality rates. These areas will require extensive investigation as to etiology, unique characteristics and better management.

Fetal Surgery

Certain lesions such as hydrocephalus, hydroureteronephrosis and diaphragmatic hernias may benefit from intrauterine correction.

Fetal Intestinal Obstruction

The fetal gastrointestinal tract (foregut, midgut and hindgut) undergoes ventral folding between 24-28 days gestation. By the 5-6th week the stomach rotates to the right and the duodenum occludes by cell proliferation. Recanalization of the duodenum occurs around the 8th wk. The midgut rotation takes place during the 6-11th week and the final peritoneal closure by 10th wk. The fetal GI tract begins ingestion and absorption of amniotic fluid by the 14th week. This fluid contributes to 17% effective nutrition; proximally obstructed gut can cause growth retardation. Fetal intestinal obstruction is caused by: failure of recanalization (duodenal atresia), vascular accidents (intestinal atresias), intrauterine volvulus, intussusception, or intraluminal obstruction (meconium ileus). Esophageal obstruction causes polyhydramnios, absent visible stomach and is related to tracheo-esophageal anomalies. Duodenal obstruction seen as two anechoic cystic masses is associated to aneuploidy (trisomy 21) and polyhydramnios. Jejuno-ileal obstruction produces dilated anechoic (fluid-filled) serpentine masses and bowel diameter of 1-2 cm. Large bowel obstruction is most often caused by meconium ileus, Hirschsprung's disease or imperforate anus. The colon assumes a large diameter and the meconium is seen echogenic during sonography. In general the method of delivery is not changed by the intrauterine diagnosis of intestinal obstruction. Timing can be affected if there is evidence of worsening intestinal ischemia (early delivery recommended after fetal lung maturity).

Fetal Abdominal Wall Defect

Most common abdominal wall defects (AWD) are gastroschisis, omphalocele and hernia of the umbilical cord. Referral to tertiary centers with available neonatal intensive care is necessary in prenatally diagnosed cases. Changing the route of delivery does not affect outcome for either defect. Omphalocele has a high incidence of associated anomalies (cardiac, neurogenic, genitourinary, skeletal, chromosomal syndromes) that are the cornerstones of mortality. Detailed search for associated anomalies, fetal echocardiogram and karyotyping should be performed always. Cesarean section is justified in large omphaloceles (> 5 cm) to avoid liver damage, sac rupture and dystocia. Gastroschisis prenatal US appearance depends on gestational age and condition of extruded bowel. Fetal karyotyping testing is less important. Intestinal atresia complicates the defect, the result of an intrauterine vascular accident. Intestinal obstruction due to atresia or luminal constriction may cause polyhydramnios, fetal growth retardation and preterm labor, findings that can be monitored with serial US. No benefit has been found in recommending routine c-section for most cases of gastroschisis. Preterm deliveries by c-section have been found to prevent bowel damage in fetus with progressive bowel dilatation and thickening, a finding that has not been corroborated by others. Abnormal US appearance of fetal bowel is associated with more bowel edema, longer operative time and a higher incidence of postoperative complications.

Chapter 11

Cosmetic Surgery

Since cosmetic surgery is seldom a necessity, the patient should carefully evaluate the surgery as well as surgeon.

Cosmetic surgery is a very specialised area of plastic surgery applied to correct undesirable features and reverse the physical signs of aging.

There are many different types of cosmetic surgery available. These include:

1. *Facial:*
   - Face Left lift (Rhytidectomy)
   - Facial implants
   - Forehead/Brow lift (Endoscopic)
   - Nasal septum surgery (Rhinoplasty)
2. Breast
   - Breast augmentation
   - Breast reduction
3. Hair
   - Hair transplant.
4. Others
   - Liposuction
   - "Tummy tuck".

FACE LIFT (RHYTIDECTOMY)

A face lift procedure is intended to provide a rejuvinated appearance. The degree of improvement depends upon the severity of the initial stages of aging of the patient.

A facelift is also known as rhytidectomy. It is not just a wrinkle removal surgery. Though deeplines and shadows are diminished, it is primarily an antigravity surgery for the lower face. It can also be a neck lift. A facelift is very beneficial whenever there is an excessive sagging of the facial or neck skin. A facelift doesn't include lifting the forehead and doesn't include lifting the forehead and does not completely raise the mild and central face.

The facelift is considered to be a major operative procedure. The type of skin, the degree of pre existing sun damage, age and the aging rate of each patient are factors that help determine the final result.

A rhytidectomy is a cosmetic surgical operation in which the loose muscles of the face and neck are tightened, and the skin is redraped and the excess trimmed.

The procedure usually requires approximately two hours. It may be performed under local anaesthesia with intravenous sedatives as required to ensure the patient's comfort, or under general anaesthesia. At the completion of the operation, drainage tubes are frequently placed beneath the skin to minimize swelling.

COMPLICATIONS

Some of the possible complications from this operation include: infection, bleeding, unequal discolouration and swelling of the ace, blistering of the skin, nerve damage causing temporary or permanent loss of sensation on the face of weakening of the facial muscles.

Breast Augmentation

Breast augmentation (or enlargement) is generally performed on women with underdeveloped breasts or on women who experienced a decrease in breast size or shape due to pregnancy or weight loss. The surgery consists of lifting the breast tissue and placing an envelop containing a soft, natural feeling implant material underneath.

Although several implants are available at the present time the implant which is used most often for augmentation purposes, is made of a silicone shell, and filled with a saline solution. Under certain conditions, silicone gel implants are used, but these are mostly used for revision surgery. The a variety of implants designs, all of which have advantages disadvantages.

Techniques

Several different methods are used for placement of the implants. An incision can be made in the crease of the lower part of breast, along the lower half of the dark skin are the nipple or in the armpit. All of these methods are design to result in minimal scarring so that the incisions are not easily detected. After the incision is made, the implant is carefully inserted either under the breast tissue beneath chest muscle. The implants are then adjusted to ideal size symmetry before the incision is sutured closed.

Breast Lift

Also known as mastopexy, the breast is performed on women who have experienced sagging or drooping of the breasts. This procedure may be done in con–junction with augmentation. Several different techni–ques can be used to correct this condition depending on the degree of sagging. Surgery consists of remov-ing excess skin from around the areola and from the bottom of the breast and rearranging skin of the breast to tighten the skin envelop. In doing surgery position of the nipple and areola can be elevated to a more natural position.

The surgery is designed to minimize scarring. Some patients who seek breast enlargement actually will need a breast the most desirable result. Your cos-metic surgeon is train help you make the proper decision.

LIPOSUCTION

Introduced in the early 1980s liposuction, is a cosmetic surgery tending cosmetic surgeons to remove stubborn fat deposits. The fatty bulges are commonly found in buttocks, knees, ankles, calves and arms.

It is natural for women, in particular, to accumulate fatty buttocks and abdomen. Some men experience enlarged breast.

Liposuction can enhance the appearance of men and women boosting their self-esteem.

Liposuction is a very popular procedure that is normally aimed at removal of excessive fat. Like all surgery, any cosmetic procedure involves risk.

Complications include uneven skin surface, especially endangered skin elasticity, bleeding, infection, discoloration, fluid accumulation under skin, numbness and scarring.

Most patients are mobile immediately after liposuction.

Index